A REFERENCE MANUAL
FOR TEACHERS
OF
DANCE EXERCISE

By JILL MAY B.E.D. Hons. Physical Education/Dance

W. FOULSHAM & CO. LIMITED
London · New York · Cape Town · Sydney

W. Foulsham & Co. Limited
Yeovil Road, Slough, Berks., England

ISBN 0-572-01472-4

Printed in Great Britain at The Bath Press, Avon

Acknowledgement

The author wishes to acknowledge the
contribution from colleagues who lectured on
'The Bodywork Dance Exercise Teacher
Training Course', on which this book is based,
and from which much of their expertise and
experience provided a valuable source of
material.

Foreword

The inspiration for writing a reference manual for dance exercise sprang from my concern over the apparent lack of information available specifically relating the body's structure and systems to the exercise class situation. It seemed that a set of guidelines was required for planning and teaching the exercise class in rather the same way as the Highway code serves the driver. In particular, there appeared to be an urgent requirement to highlight the need for safe standards of teaching in exercise.

In the process of setting up and organising a teacher training course, I have collected much relevant information in this context, and so it seemed an obvious step to pass this on in the interests of raising safety standards within the teaching profession. It is hoped that the information provided in this book will help all teachers and aspiring teachers of dance exercise to promote the message of health-related fitness through exercise in the safest possible way.

Jill May

Contents

Introduction

To assume the role of exercise teacher presents each of us who achieve that status with an awesome responsibility. Clearly, the exercise teacher sets herself up as an exemplary model of a particular lifestyle: a lifestyle which demonstrates that exercise is good for people.

As advocates of a gospel that preaches 'fitness' as a way of life, we are in the business of positively promoting health. This puts us into the category of practitioners of alternative medicine, proposing an alternative lifestyle to that which is sedentary and inactive. We are, after all, attempting to preserve health and, so doing, we have a great responsibility to ensure that we administer that medicine safely and wisely.

The following chapters are intended as a guide to all qualified teachers of exercise who wish to uphold high standards of safety and maintain a high reputation as caring, responsible instructors. The recent interest in fitness and health has motivated many people, who may themselves be highly proficient in exercise skills, towards ambitions to teach those skills to others. Unfortunately, an unqualified instructor can do more harm than good, and reports of injuries caused to people attending poorly tutored classes have resulted in a reaction against aerobic exercise from the media and the general public. At present, opinion on the value of exercise seems to fall between two extremes: the experts who warn that 'exercise can damage your health', and those who advise that 'exercise is good for you'.

It is most important that we, as teachers, are very well informed and can clearly appreciate and evaluate the good points and the pitfalls in order to present our case for the benefits of exercise in contributing to a healthy lifestyle.

In answer to the question 'Why exercise'? we need to be aware of what the terms 'health' and 'fitness' imply. The World Health Organisation (WHO) defines good health as "a complete feeling of mental and physical well-being – not merely the absence of disease and infirmity, but the presence of vigour, vitality and social well being – a zest for living." Similarly, WHO defines physical fitness as "the ability to carry out daily tasks with vigour and alertness, without undue fatigue and with ample reserve energy to enjoy leisure pursuits and meet unforeseen emergencies."

Such qualities as those defined by WHO may easily be taken for granted. Good health is fundamental to our existence and enjoyment of life, yet often it is not appreciated until something goes wrong. Unfortunately, there is evidence to suggest that we do need to be concerned about the adverse effects of sedentary lifestyles and the various forms of abuse to which we voluntarily subject our bodies, or which are forced upon them by our working environment.

Twentieth-century man, unlike his predecessor who was an active mammal, leads a comparatively sedentary life. Undoubtedly, the maximum physical capacity of most individuals has decreased significantly. To keep the body in good working order the muscles and joints need a combination of anaerobic exercise to strengthen, aerobic exercise to tone, and stretching exercise to keep them supple.

A thorough understanding of anatomy and physiology, as they relate to the body during exercise activity, is fundamental to any instructor's basic working knowledge. The chapter on the cardiovascular system (p. 27) illustrates how fitness is attained through increasing the efficiency of the heart, lungs and circulatory system.

Heart disease is still the greatest killer disease in the UK, and one of its major causes is clogging of the arteries. The heart is a muscular organ which responds to exercise. In the same way as other muscles it may enlarge and strengthen as a result of exercise. Other major risk factors in the onset of heart disease are smoking, raised blood pressure (hypertension), increased fat in the blood (cholesterol), obesity and stress. Each of these may be an operative factor in the production of fatty deposits in the coronary arteries.

Fitness, as a lifestyle, encourages good diet. Those who develop a positive programme of exercise as part of their lifestyle are more likely to consider carefully what they eat. Exercise certainly produces a feeling of well-being which in turn must reduce the levels of stress induced by the strains and aggravations of modern living. Studies have shown that hypertension may be beneficially affected by exercise. Excess alcohol consumption and smoking are both voluntary activities which have adverse effects on health. Recent research suggests that exercise may modify the risk factors for heart disease, and in some cases may even prevent their development. Exercise is probably the best way to redress the balance and to combat the excesses of modern living. Combined with a good diet, minimal alcohol and no smoking, exercise definitely improves the cardiovascular system.

Given such an impressive array of benefits from exercise there would seem to be no reason for hesitation in the adoption of the new fitness-oriented lifestyle. Indeed, in a very few years the fitness boom has encouraged a great many to take up some form of exercise programme in their leisure time. We are all in a position to choose the type of exercise programme which best suits our needs. However, with so much conflicting advice from both medical experts and the media, and with so many commercial organisations geared to provide a service, it is no wonder that we sometimes become confused and misdirected.

Most problems with exercise programmes have arisen as a result of participation in strenuous aerobic dance exercise routines, particularly those involving prolonged periods of jogging. The resulting high number of injuries sustained has spread alarm and consternation and given rise to conflicting advice. The great majority of such injuries can be avoided provided sufficient care is taken by the class instructor to prevent any potentially harmful situation arising. The responsibility for the safety and care of the class lies entirely with the instructor. It is her duty to be fully aware of the risks involved in exercise, and to conduct the exercise programme with the safety of each individual in mind. The chapter on Safety Considerations in the Exercise Programme sets out guidelines for injury prevention (p. 37).

The design of an exercise programme relies on an understanding of the logical progression of ideas for movement in a properly balanced sequence. This, combined with interesting and creative material for the actual body action, contributes to the creation of a lively and stimulating class atmosphere within a balanced framework. The chapters on class design, choreography and dance illustrate ways of achieving this harmony.

The well-structured exercise programme should provide the opportunity for healthy enjoyment while exercising, with minimal risk of injury to participants. The opportunities to participate in exercise need to be both convenient and in pleasant circumstances, to encourage constant attendance. Man is by nature a lazy beast and motivation to sustain fitness may be erratic. As instructors and exemplary models we are helping to effect a change in attitudes towards personal health and well-being, for which each individual must be directly-responsible. Ill health can be caused by over-indulgence and unwise behaviour. Smoking, obesity, alcohol and drug dependence are all major contributors to ill health, yet the problems they cause are preventable if we each take positive action to improve our health through a radical change in lifestyle.

Instructors are the agents of change – they will modify public behaviour and encourage better standards of health.

Major bones

Major muscles

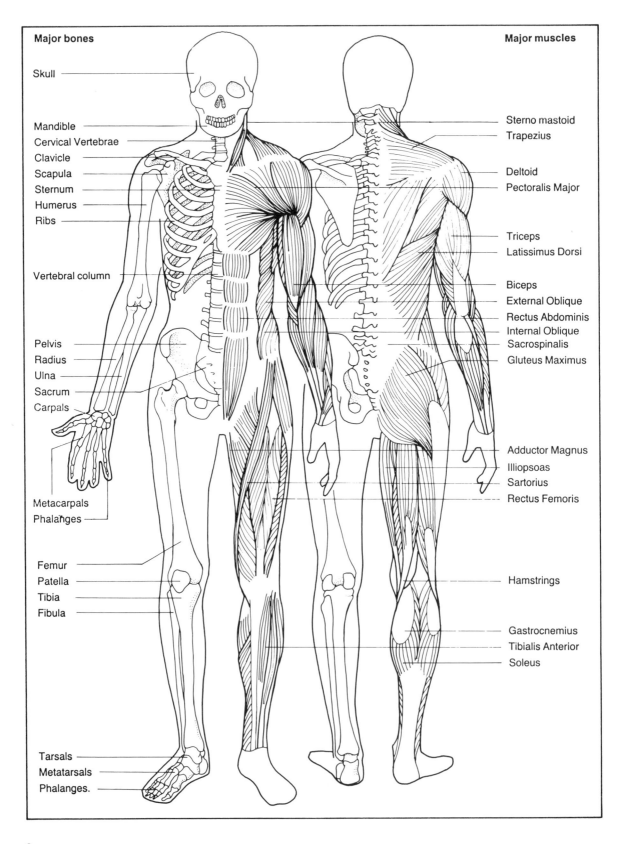

Skull

Mandible
Cervical Vertebrae
Clavicle
Scapula
Sternum
Humerus
Ribs

Vertebral column

Pelvis
Radius
Ulna
Sacrum
Carpals

Metacarpals
Phalanges

Femur
Patella
Tibia
Fibula

Tarsals
Metatarsals
Phalanges.

Sterno mastoid
Trapezius

Deltoid
Pectoralis Major

Triceps
Latissimus Dorsi

Biceps
External Oblique
Rectus Abdominis
Internal Oblique
Sacrospinalis
Gluteus Maximus

Adductor Magnus
Illiopsoas
Sartorius
Rectus Femoris

Hamstrings

Gastrocnemius
Tibialis Anterior
Soleus

8

Anatomy

Anatomy is the study of the structure of the body, in effect its appearance, composition and function.

The study of anatomy in relation to exercise contributes to an informed understanding of the body parts and their possible range of movement, so that we as teachers of movement may design appropriate exercise programmes.

The language of anatomy can be complicated. It is necessary to know and refer to some of the terms relating to body structure, positions and motion in order fully to understand the relationship between the body parts, and how this may determine the way in which the body performs movement. This aspect of anatomy is called musculoskeletal anatomy, and concerns the joints, connective tissue and muscles.

Musculoskeletal Anatomy

The skeleton consists of a framework of bones put together with joints. The skeleton gives the body its general shape, supports the body and protects the organs inside it.

Muscles are a collection of fibres which are grouped in bundles. Each bundle is wrapped in a protective sheath which holds it together. Muscles are connected to bone by tendons.

Terminology of Principal Movements

Movement of the body is brought about by the action of muscles on the bones, which act as levers. The principal movements achieved by the muscles at the various joints are:

Flexion: bending or decreasing the angle between two bones (closing a joint).

Extension: stretching/straightening, or increasing the angle between two bones, (opening a joint).

Hyperextension: extension carried beyond the normal anatomical position.

Abduction: moving the body part away from the centre line. (e.g., raising an arm to the side.)

Adduction: bringing the body part back to the centre line (lowering an arm to the side).

Supination: turning/rotating the body part upwards and outwards (e.g., hand, palm up).

Pronation: turning/rotating the body part downwards and inwards (e.g., hand, palm down).

Rotation: pivoting the body part inwards or outwards around a long axis (e.g., rolling the head).

Circumduction: a complete circular motion of the body part (e.g., circling the arm at the shoulder).

Eversion: turning the body part outwards (e.g., foot, sole out).

Inversion: turning the body part inwards (e.g., foot, sole in).

Dorsiflexion: turning the toes up towards the shins.

Plantarflexion: pointing the toes.

In relation to these movements, and to anatomy in general, the following positional terms may also be used:

Anterior: in front or forward.

Posterior: behind or towards the back.

Medial: near the mid-line of the body.

Lateral: to the side, away from the mid-line

Superior: above, or towards the top of the head.

Inferior: below, or down from the top of the head.

The Skeletal System

The skeletal system, or skeleton, is the bony framework of the body, and is composed of cartilage and bone.

CARTILAGE (gristle) is an elastic connective tissue found in adults principally at the joints between bones. It allows the body part to be flexible. Cartilage may cover the ends of bones to reduce friction in a joint (articular cartilage), or may be found in the centre of a joint where it takes the form of discs (e.g., in the spine).

BONE At birth the bones are extremely flexible because they are composed largely of cartilage. They gradually grow more rigid with age as true bone is formed. Compositionally, the bones are about 50 percent water and other fluids, and 50 percent solid material.

There are two types of bone tissue. Compact hard bone forms the surface layer of all bones and the whole shaft of the long bones (arms, legs and ribs). Cancellate bone is spongy and is found inside compact bone in wrists, ankles, shoulder, pelvis and skull.

Four types of bones occur in the skeleton and the relationship between their structure and function is shown in the table.

Structure and Function of the Four Bone Types

Structure	Function of the four bone types
Long bones:– arms, legs and ribs	… Act as levers to move the body; ribs move chest during respiration
Short bones:– wrist and ankles	… give *strength* and *mobility* to joints.
Flat bones:– shoulder blades, pelvis and skull	… Provide *protection* for internal organs.
Irregular bones:– vertebrae, facial bones	… Provide *support* for the body

Functions of the Skeleton

The functions of the skeleton can be summarised, as follows:

1. Support and strength. Without the supportive function of bone, the body would be floppy and shapeless.

2. Attachment for muscle. The skeleton is jointed to allow movement, which is brought about by the action of muscles attached to the bones.

3   The bones act as
        ent to occur.

4. Protec..   ..y parts. In particular
the skull protec..   .e brain, the rib cage
protects the lungs and heart, and the pelvis
protects the abdominal organs.

Joints

A joint, or articulation, is formed where two
or more bones come together. Joints allow the
body to move and can be classified according
to their type of mobility as freely movable
(synovial joints), semi-movable
(intervertebral joints) and immovable joints.
Joints are made up of bones covered in
articular cartilage, encased in a capsule
consisting of an outer layer of collagen fibres,
reinforced with strong protective ligaments,
and an inner layer of synovial membrane.
Within the inner layer the joint is surrounded
by synovial fluid, which acts as a lubricant.

    The thickness of the cartilage is normally
dependent on the amount of stress to which
the joint is subjected. The cartilage is able to
absorb substances from the synovial fluid and
swell temporarily.

Exercise note:–
After warming up in exercise, there is a
temporary thickening of the articular
cartilage, and the synovial membrane
stimulates the release of synovial fluid,
lubricating the joints.

Instructor's safety check:

1. Prolonged training can cause a permanent thickening
of the cartilage.

2. Severe or uneven stress can wear the cartilage away
and restrict the movement of the joint.

    The muscles are attached to the bones at the
joints by strong *tendons* of tough connecting
tissue composed largely of collagen fibres.

Ligaments are similar to tendons, but connect
bone to bone and act as stabilizers reinforcing
the joint. They are assisted by the muscle and
the actual structure of the joint.

Exercise note:–
The degree of elasticity in the ligament
depends on the joint itself, sex, age and
physical fitness of the individual.

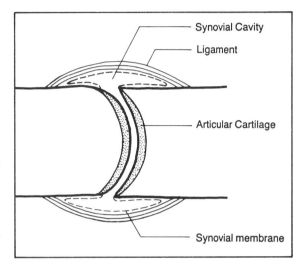

Synovial Cavity
Ligament
Articular Cartilage
Synovial membrane

Instructor's safety check

1. Exercises performed too quickly may overstretch the
ligaments and cause them to lose their elasticity.

2. Ballistic bouncing movements place a direct strain on
the ligaments, leading to permanent stretching and
joint instability.

Freely movable (synovial) joints

These joints have the widest range of
movement. The amount of freedom of
movement in a particular joint is determined
by the way in which it can be used, and the
limiting factors are dependent upon the shape
of the bone ends meeting at the joint (e.g.,
flexion of the elbow is limited by the ulna
coming against the humerus), strong bands of
ligaments, and soft parts, e.g., muscles,
coming into contact.

Hinge joints, e.g., elbow and knee, give a wide range of movement in one plane. Their principal movements are extension and flexion.

Condyloid join _ _ _ ive movement in _ _ _ _ _ al movements _ _ _ _ _), extension (_ _ _ _ _ on (Rotation in _ _ _ _ _ n outward), pr _ _ _ _ supination (Ro _

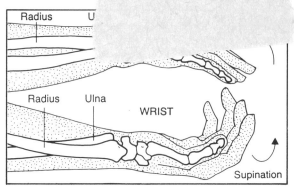

Ball and socket joints, e.g., hip and shoulders, give movement in three planes and allow rotation, making them the most freely moveable. Their principal movements are flexion, extension, hyperextension, abduction, adduction, rotation (medial and lateral) and circumduction.

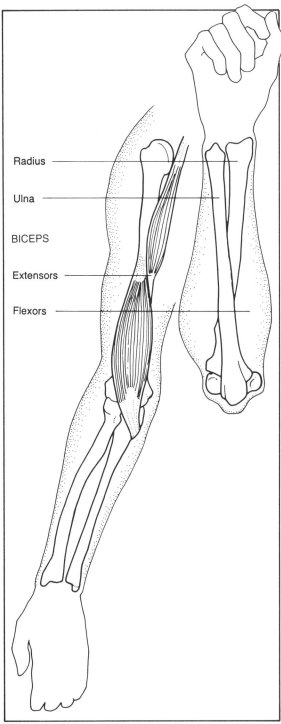

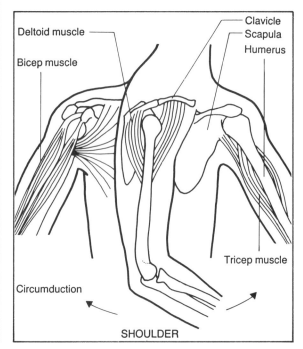

The hip has a wonderful range of movement and mobility is important. Overstretching in this area will, however, produce hypermobility to an unsafe degree.

Hypermobility is classified as:
(a) Hyperextension of joints such as the knee or elbow beyond 10 degrees.
(b) Passive extension of the metacarpophalangeal joints (finger knuckles) beyond 90 degrees.
(c) Placing the palms of the hands flat on the floor with knees straight from a standing position.
(d) Touching the thumb to the underside of the wrist or forearm.

The range of motion in active extension of the hip joint (i.e., taking the leg forward or backward yourself) is between 10 and 15 degrees. Passive extension (as in the leg being lifted by another person) in the forward-backward plane can be safe for up to 30 degrees of hyperextension.

Activities such as the 'splits' go beyond 30 degrees and become forced extension. This is unsafe hyperextension and leads to tearing of the iliofemoral ligament at the front of the hip. Injury to this important 'stay' of the hip joint leads to instability of the joint itself and can be extremely damaging.

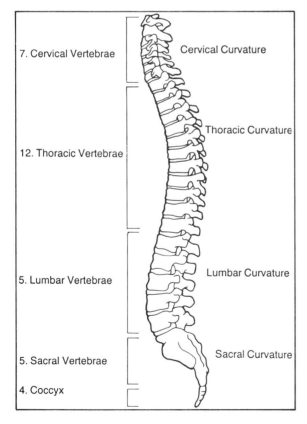

7. Cervical Vertebrae — Cervical Curvature

12. Thoracic Vertebrae — Thoracic Curvature

5. Lumbar Vertebrae — Lumbar Curvature

5. Sacral Vertebrae — Sacral Curvature

4. Coccyx

Semimoveable (Intervertebral) Joints

These joints are separated by discs of cartilage, which allow only slight movement. The relatively large number of intervertebral joints gives the vertebral column its flexibility.

The vertebral column, or spine, is divided into five regions: the *cervical spine* contains 7 vertebrae in the neck and shoulder; the *thoracic spine* contains 12 vertebrae; the *lumbar spine* contains 5 vertebrae in the small of the back; the *sacral region* contains 5 vertebrae fused together to form the sacrum in the pelvic area; and the *coccyx* contains 4 vertebrae fused together in the tail bone.

1. Where pelvic bones join the spine is a synovial joint, but care must be taken not to move it *beyond its normal range of motion*. Slight sacroiliac joint play is essential for transference of weight, as in normal walking. The pelvis, which consists of a large articulated arch (two sacroiliac joints and the pubic joint) is liable to displacement, pubic joint instability and sacroiliac strain are common problems which can occur from overstretching in this area, a severe blow or having one leg slightly shorter than the other. This tilt shifts the body weight carried through the spine to the pelvis and can lead to locking of one sacroiliac joint. Activities which involve bending with twisting can produce locking of the joint and pain in the groin, the joint itself or deep in the buttock.
2. Excessive jogging or jumping on a poor floor surface may result in injury to the lower back jarring discs.

Curvatures are present in four regions of the spine. The thoracic and sacral curvatures are present at birth, while the cervical and lumbar curvatures develop as the child matures.

The vertebral column's function:

1. Provides a firm support to the body.
2. Intervertebral discs act as shock absorbers when the weight of the body is moved in running and jumping, so the brain and spinal cord are protected from shocks and jarring.

3. Curvatures give flexibility and enable the column to move without breaking.
4. Supports the weight of the body – overweight and pregnant people often complain of backache.
5. Provides surfaces for the attachment of muscles.
6. Acts as a prop for the rib cage and pelvis, which contain and protect the vulnerable body organs (e.g., heart, lungs, reproductive organs).
7. Provides attachment for the ribs.

Immovable Joints

The fibrous joints (sutures) between the flat bones of the skull are immovable.

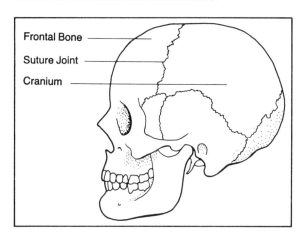

Frontal Bone

Suture Joint

Cranium

Joint Movement

The movement of a joint is brought about by muscular contraction or relaxation. Movement is limited by the shape of the joint, and by connective tissues such as ligaments, tendons and the formation of the capsule surrounding the joint. The possible movements at particular joints are shown in the table.

The two characteristics of a joint are mobility, i.e., *allowing a wide range of movement,* and stability, i.e., *allowing a limited range of movement.* Both qualities are necessary, but in planning an exercise we should be aware that overextension of mobility may damage the structures which give the joint its stability. For example, hinge joints such as the knee are designed for limited flexion and extension.

Exercise note:–

Avoid exercises that twist the knee, move it from side to side or exaggerate its normal range of flexion and extension.

Instructor's safety check

A joint and its structures may be harmed when:
1. Movements go beyond a desirable range of motion.
2. Movements are performed incorrectly and place great stress upon a joint.
3. Movements are performed too fast without proper body control.

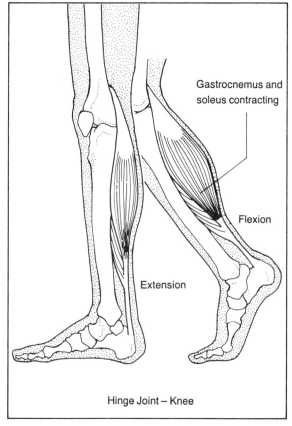

Gastrocnemius and soleus contracting

Flexion

Extension

Hinge Joint – Knee

Possible Joint Movement

Spine	Flexion Extension Hyperextension Lateral flexion (side bending) Rotation (minimal)
Pelvis	Forward Backward Lateral
Hip Shoulder	Flexion Extension Hyperextension Abduction Adduction Rotation (medial/lateral) Circumduction
Knee	Flexion Extension
Ankle	Dorsiflexion Plantarflexion Inversion (rotation inward) Eversion (rotation outward)
Wrist	Flexion Extension Supination (rotation outward) Pronation (rotation inward)

Muscular System

The main characteristic of muscle is that it is elastic and contractile. Even at rest there is a slight tension called 'tone'. Muscle is composed of short and long fibres grouped together in bundles surrounded by a sheath of connective tissue. There are three types of muscle tissue.

Cardiac muscle: found in the heart, this type of muscle does not tire easily unless the heart rate is greatly increased over a long period or there is insufficient rest between muscle contractions.

Involuntary muscle: these muscles are not under direct control, e.g., those in the digestive system.

Voluntary or skeletal muscle: these muscles are directly responsible for body movement. They are stimulated by nerves to contract and thereby initiate movement. The strength of the muscle contraction depends on the number of fibres stimulated.

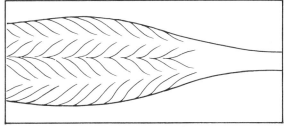

Many short Fibres into several strands of tendon = very strong muscle.

Once stimulated, each muscle fibre contracts *totally* or not at all, with a brief latent period after relaxation, before contraction can occur again.

In lifting a weight the appropriate number of fibres will contract fully, while those not needed remain inactive. When the weight is increased, all the fibres may be stimulated to contract fully, at which point the individual's 'work limit' would be reached. The response of the muscle is related to the demand made upon it. Therefore, to maintain their efficiency muscles must have sufficient demand placed upon them.

Exercise note:–
Normal healthy resting muscle has firmness, resilience and shape, i.e., good muscle tone. This can be achieved through regular exercise. Firm muscles in good tone protect the joints. A diminished muscle tone leaves the joints prone to strain. Illness or increasing age may contribute to a lessening of muscle tone, while excessive muscle tone, as a result of overtraining, leads to abnormal state of muscle tension.

Exercise rule:–

For efficient working of the muscle, *relaxation* should always follow *contraction*.

Muscle Action

Skeletal muscle may be attached directly to bone, by fibrous tendon to the bone, or to the fibrous tissue of other muscles. The major muscle groups are shown in the table. Muscles generally work in pairs and act like wires pulling on the bone. When one of the muscle pair contracts to pull the bone forward, the other will act to pull it back.

Within the pair one can be identified as prime mover or *agonist*, i.e., the muscle group performing the action, and the other as secondary mover or *antagonist*, i.e., the muscle group performing the opposite movement to the agonist. The agonist contracts (flexor), while the antagonist is stretched (extensor).

The central nervous system is responsible for maintaining a perfect balance between the agonist and antagonist. The mass of tiny filaments which make up the muscle fibres respond to received messages – nerve impulses – and move toward each other to contract and away from each other to relax. Sometimes a group of muscles will work to hold one part of the body in position whilst another part moves. These muscles are known as *fixators*. For example, in abdominal exercise the abdominal muscles sometimes act as fixators while the legs bicycle.

Exercise note:–

When a muscle contracts it generally moves the less stable part of the skeletal structure toward the more stable part.

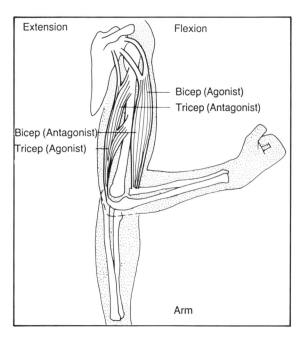

Arm

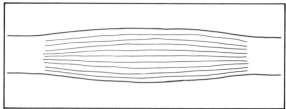

1. Muscle relaxed

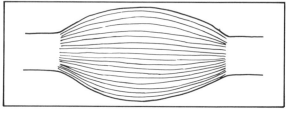

2. Muscle contracted

Major Muscle Groups

Body Area	Flexors	Extensors	Abductors	Adductors
Spine and Trunk	Rectus Abdominis	Sacrospinalis	–	–
Hip	Iliopsoas Rectus femoris Sartorious	Gluteal Muscles Hamstrings	Iliotibial band	Adductor magnus, brevis and longus
Knee	Hamstrings	Quadriceps	–	–
Ankle	Tibialis anterior	Gastrocnemius Soleus	Evertors	Invertors
Shoulder, Chest Upper back	Pectoralis major and minor	Latissimus dorsi Trapezius	Deltoid Serratus anterior	Pectoralis major and minor Latissimus dorsi
Elbow	Biceps	Triceps	–	–

Muscles move joints where they cross them and may cross one, two or more joints. The action of the muscle may therefore cause movement in several joints at once.

Instructor's safety check

1. In a two joint muscle exercise the stretch may only be felt in one area, or the wrong one, so that advice may be needed on adjustment of body position to feel the stretch correctly.
2. Warm muscle works better than cold ones.
3. Adequate preparation and stretching of the muscle before contraction will help it to function more efficiently.
4. A tired muscle works less efficiently and is prone to strain.
5. Exercise clothing should be loose and non-restrictive to allow blood to circulate freely.

Skeletal muscle contraction can be *static* or dynamic. During a static or *isometric* contraction there is no movement in the joint over which the muscle crosses. Exercises using isometric muscle contraction are those requiring balance or stationary positions. Dynamic or *isotonic* muscle contraction requires a changing of muscle length. In the first phase the muscle may shorten in a concentric contraction, causing the joint to move (e.g., lifting the arm). In the second phase the muscle lengthens in an eccentric contraction (e.g., lowering the arm).

During the exercise, the nervous system increases the rate of the heart beat, dilates small blood vessels in the working muscles and increases the rate and depth of breathing. The sweat glands produce more sweat in anticipation of heat production during activity. Muscles in the digestive tract slow down or cease their activity for a while.

Regular, controlled breathing during strong muscle work should be encouraged. In most cases breathing in during the relaxation period and out during the effort period, is desirable.

All strong muscle work should be interspersed with more relaxed stretching exercise, which acts in a compensatory manner. Time must be allowed for an adequate 'warm down' period.

Programme Design

In exercise analysis the instructor should be fully conversant with:–
the possible movements of the joint
what limitations are imposed on the joint
which major muscle groups are involved
additional factors affecting movement in that area of the body
the emphasis of the exercise, either toward strengthening and conditioning, or toward mobility and flexibility.

When preparing the exercise programme it is useful to name the exercise, identify the primary joints involved in the exercise, name their movements or positions and be clear about the purpose of the exercise. For example:

Body Part	Name/Description	Purpose/Special instruction
Hamstring	Low Bounces	Relax thighs – weight forward
and	Hamstring Stretch	Stretch Hamstring – slowly smoothly
Quadriceps	Single leg stretch Right and left in turn	Quadricep stretch – weight over support knee Stretched knee straight
Basic Level Hamstring	Low bounces	as before
Stretch	Hamstring stretch	As before

The joint movement possible, limitations, muscle groups involved and additional qualifying factors are charted on pp 19-22.

Reference charts of Joint and Muscle Movements

Joint	Possible Movements	Limited By	Major Muscle Groups	Notes
Neck Atlanto-occipital: Special joint between skull and atlas, i.e., 1st cervical vertebra	Nodding	Surrounding structures shape of actual bones	Sternomastoid – Flexes neck Splenius Semispinalis Capitis Sacrospinalis-extend neck	Two sides of muscle acting together
Atlanto-Axial: Synovial Pivot	Turning Head takes place between atlas and axis (1st and 2nd cervical vertebrae	Surrounding structures shape of vertebrae	Sternomastoid Splenius Semispinalis Capitis	Action of one side of muscle
	Lateral flexion takes place below atlas and axis in cervical vertebrae, as does flexion and extension		Sternomastoid Splenius As for 'Nodding'	Action of one side of muscle

Joint	Possible Movements	Limited By	Major Muscle Groups	Notes
Shoulder: Synovial, Ball and socket	Flexion	Ligaments of shoulder joint opposite muscle group	Deltoid Pectoral muscle	Full shoulder movement relies on range of movement at shoulder joint and girdle
	Extension	Ligaments and opposite muscle group	Deltoid Latissimus Dorsi Teres Major	
	Abduction	Head of Humerus contacting bony arch of shoulder girdle. varies in individuals. Arm then raised above head by moving shoulder girdle	Deltoid Supraspinatus	Shoulder joint is very shallow, head of humerus large so muscles very important in keeping region secure. More liable to dislocation than any other joint
	Adduction	Contact of arm with body opposite muscle group and ligaments.	Pectoral muscle – in front Latissimus Dorsi – behind Subscapularis Teres major	
	Rotation Circumduction (arm circling)	Ligaments and muscles around joint combined movement of shoulder joint and girdle – limitations as for those of both joints.	Most of muscles attached to shoulder region brought into action	
Shoulder Girdle 1. Sterno-clavicular (clavicle glides with sternum): Synovial 2. Clavicular-scapular – (clavicle and shoulder blade): Synovial Shoulder blades on chest wall	The Shoulder Blades move on chest wall and can move vertically (hunch and lower) Abduction: Move round chest wall Adduction: Shoulder blades move towards spine Rotation of lower end of scapulae up and out/down and in when arms lifted above head	Size of articular surfaces and available freedom of scapulae (shoulder blades)	Muscles of scapulae produce movement	Movement of shoulder girdle can be independent of shoulder joint

Joint	Possible Movements	Limited By	Major Muscle Groups	Notes
Elbow: Synovial, hinge	Flexion	Limit of articular areas, ligaments and opposite muscle, contact of lower and upper arm	Biceps Brachialis Flexor muscles of forearm	
	Extension	Locking of joint by ulna into humerus	Triceps Anconeus	
	Lateral movement	None – shape of bony surfaces and strong ligaments		
Forearm: Synovial, Pivot	Supination: palm up Pronation: palm down	Radius pivots in a circle of ligament attached to ulna. Lower end of radius crosses ulna taking hand with it.	Biceps Supinator Pronators	

Trunk

There are two types of joint between vertebrae. Between two vertebral bodies, the joint is semi-movable and weight bearing. Between small articular facets on vertebral arches, joints are synovial and gliding: These determine direction and degree of movement at specific level of spine.

Joint	Notes
Between Vertebral bodies: semi-movable	Fibro-cartilaginous disc is between bodies. Strong ligaments run length of vertebral column in front and behind (Latter within vertebral canal). Movement due to compression of disc: in front to flex spine, behind to extend it, at sides to flex laterally. Thickness of disc and opposing ligaments limit movement. Deep spinal muscles protect spinal column
Between articular Facets on arches of vertebrae: synovial gliding	Different planes of movement possible in different areas of spine, owing to direction of facets. Range of movement at one joint very small, but range of spinal movement considerable overall.

Possible movement of trunk	Major Muscle Groups	Notes
Flexion: Forward movement	Rectus Abdominis (Band down centre of abdomen)	Controls pelvic tilt and therefore assists in flattening lumbar curve.
	External oblique (right and left sides of abdomen)	Right side of muscle twists to left and vice versa.
	Internal Oblique (right and left sides of abdomen) [In sitting up and taking left elbow to right knee, left external oblique and right internal oblique do twist at same time also flexing trunk with rectus abdominis]	Right side of muscle twists to right and vice versa. Transversus Abdominis with Obliques and Rectus Abdominis helps hold abdomen flat
Extension: Backward movement of spine of head and neck	Quadratus Lumborum Sacrospinalis – includes three spinal muscles also inclines head and neck Splenius (also helps in side bending and twisting)	Important posturally Tone in this muscle helps head and neck posturally
Lateral Flexion: side bending	Action of one side only – Rectus Abdominis, Quadratus Lumborum, Sacrospinalis (Obliques with rotation as above)	
Rotation: Twisting	Obliques Postural muscles lying under Sacrospinalis aid in rotation and lateral flexion.	

Joint	Possible Movements	Limited By	Major Muscle Groups	Notes
Hip: Synovial/ freely movable, ball and socket	Flexion	Opposite muscle groups, especially hamstrings if legs straight. Contact of soft parts if knee bent	Hip Flexors Iliopsoas Psoas Major Pectineus Iliacus Tensor fasciae latae Sartorius Rectus femoris	very important in maintenance of upright posture of trunk in standing, walking, etc.
	Extension	Ligaments at front of hip joint. After little movement back arches and there is movement in lower spine	Hip Extensors Gluteus Maximus Hamstrings (Biceps femoris Semi-membranosis Semi-tendinosus)	
	Abduction	Tension of opposite muscle group and contact of tip of femur with edge of socket	Abductors Gluteus medius, Gluteus minimus ilio – tibial band – Tensor fasciae latae	
	Adduction	By opposite muscle group and contact with other leg	Adductors Pectineus Adductor longus – magnus – brevis Gracilis	
	Rotation: outwards or inwards	Opposite muscle groups and strong ligaments	A combination of some of the above muscles e.g. Gluteus maximus – outward rotator. Iliopsoas – inward rotator	
	Circling	Combination of all movements with corresponding limitations		

Joint	Possible Movements	Limited By	Major Muscle Groups	Notes
Knee: synovial, hinge	Flexion	Short quadriceps muscles Contact of soft parts, i.e. calf muscle with thigh,	Hamstrings Gracilis Sartorius Popliteus Gastrocnemius (double bellied muscle) Soleus (flat underneath) Plantaris (ends at Achilles tendon)	Very powerful muscle. Gives force in running, jumping, hopping, skipping
	Extension	Limit of articular surfaces. Tight hamstrings if hip is flexed. Can extend knee little more by pulling up knee cap	Quadriceps – Rectus femoris Vastus lateralis Vastus intermedius Vastus medialis	
	Lateral movement	None. Prevented by very strong ligaments on inner and outer sides of joint		
	Rotation outward and inwards	No voluntary rotation		Need strong and effective knee, as combined functions of weight bearing and locomotion place considerable stress and strain on it. Ligaments and muscle tendons (cont)

provide strong support. Joint surfaces between tibia and femur protected and cushioned by cartilage

Joint	Possible Movements	Limited By	Major Muscle Groups	Notes
Ankle: Synovial, Hinge	(Dorsi) Flexion: foot pulled up towards shin	Short Achilles tendon shape of joint surface	Tibialis Anterior Long extensors of toes	
	Plantar Flexion (extension: pointing foot down)	By tendons and ligaments in front of ankle joint	Gastrocnemius with Soleus. Tibialis Posterior Long flexors of toes	
	Lateral	None		
	Rotation	None – see joints of foot for apparent rotation		

Joint	Possible Movements	Limited By	Major Muscle Groups	Notes
Foot Mid-Foot: Synovial-gliding, several small bones involved	Inversion (turning in)	Pure movement only if ankle flexed, limited by ligaments and tendons on outer side of ankle and foot, smallness of joint surfaces	Tibialis Anterior. Long flexors of toes. Tibialis posterior	
	Eversion (turning out)	Limitations on inner side of foot and ankle	Long extensor of toes Peroneus	
Between all small bones adjoined to one another:– Synovial-gliding		Small bones form gliding joints and help form arch of foot, which is supported by ligaments and muscles on sole	Peroneus Tibialis anterior Tibialis posterior (Maintain arches)	Support and propulsion are two functions of the foot. Therefore, muscles must be strong. Therefore, must be exercised especially on days when tend not to walk very far
Toes: Synovial, Hinge	Flexion:- curling up toes	Limit of articular areas – short muscle tendons	Long flexors of toes	Cramp easily
	Extension: turning up toes	Small articulations Tendons on sole	Long extensors of toes	
	Foot circling	This is combination of movements at ankle joint and joints of mid-foot – flexion and extension at ankle, inversion and eversion at mid-foot		

Biomechanics

Biomechanics, as the word implies, is the application of the principles of mechanics and engineering (in which are involved systems of leverage) to anatomy and physiology. Since the body moves by using a system of levers, we can apply the principles of mechanics and engineering to the human body in motion.

Exercise note:–

The study of biomechanics enables the instructor to understand more clearly the techniques of performance in exercise, and through close observation to be aware of errors in technique which may occur in individual movements, and so allow for correction. More important, it should also provide a basis for the instructor to design a safe programme of exercise, tailored to the needs of the participants in an exercise class.

Levers

A lever is defined as a *straight bar* which turns or pivots around a fixed point, or *fulcrum,* if acted upon by opposing forces.

In the body the *joint* is the fulcrum, in that it acts as a pivot about which the movement takes place, while the *bone* is the lever. The opposing forces acting upon the lever are resistance, which is the *weight* to be moved (i.e., body part or limb), and force which is the *effort* or power moving the weight (i.e., the muscle group contracting). The distance between the weight (resistance) and the fulcrum is called the weight arm. The distance between the effort (force) and the fulcrum is called the effort arm.

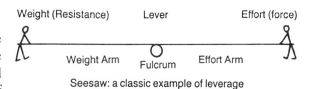

Weight (Resistance) Lever Effort (force)

Weight Arm Fulcrum Effort Arm

Seesaw: a classic example of leverage

There must be sufficient effort at one end to move the lever and offset the weight at the other. The greater the distance between the effort (muscle) and fulcrum (joint), i.e., the longer the effort arm, the less power is needed to move the weight (limb).

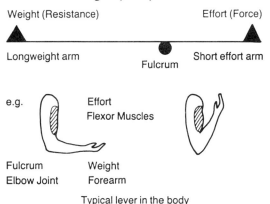

Weight (Resistance) Effort (Force)

Longweight arm Fulcrum Short effort arm

e.g. Effort
Flexor Muscles

Fulcrum Weight
Elbow Joint Forearm

Typical lever in the body

Most levers in the body have a longer distance between the limb (weight) to be moved and the joint (fulcrum) than between the muscle attachment (effort) and the joint (fulcrum). As a result they require more effort to function. They do, however, have the advantage of giving speed and a wide range of movement to the human body.

The system of leverage in the body is thus designed with short effort arms and long weight arms, which means that the muscular system must be strong to supply the necessary power for movement, particularly in strenuous activity and exercise.

Exercise note:–

Most exercise classes will consist of groups of participants who vary in size, shape, and level of fitness and ability. This can result in underworking or overworking of individuals within the same class if the instructor expects everyone to work at the same level.

Instructor's safety check

It is possible, with an understanding of leverage systems, to teach the class members to make small adjustments in the exercises – either down to lessen the exercise effect, or up to increase it.

1. Adjustment of *resistance* (weight)
   Increasing the weight i.e., adding hand weights to the movement, will increase the workload and maximise the exercise.

2. Adjustment of *force*, i.e., strength and speed of muscular contraction. This may be effected by changing the speed of the movement. Sometimes performing an exercise more slowly is more demanding and requires greater muscular control.

3. Adjustment of *distance* (weight arm).
   Shortening the length of the weight arm (distance of the limb from the joint) will modify the intensity of the exercise, while lengthening it will increase its difficulty. There will be a greater range of movement at the end of a long lever. However, using a short lever sometimes means that the speed of the movement can be increased.

Programme design

This principle of adjustment of exercise can be applied to all sections of the aerobic dance exercise programme where progression is required over a period of time. The instructor will need to be fully aware of the needs of individual participants, in order to advise on the adjustment required to increase or decrease the intensity of the exercise throughout the programme. This ensures that the instructor has control over the activity of the class and contributes to the safety of movements within the programme.

Examples of adjustment

Lengthening the distance of the weight arm from the fulcrum to increase the intensity of the exercise can be introduced gradually, as shown.

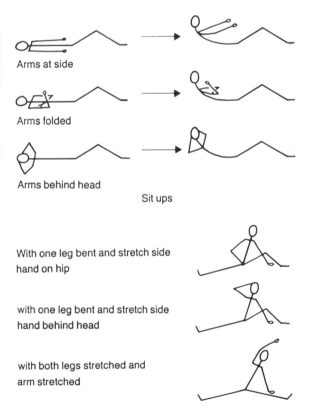

Arms at side

Arms folded

Arms behind head

Sit ups

With one leg bent and stretch side hand on hip

with one leg bent and stretch side hand behind head

with both legs stretched and arm stretched

Side Stretch Floor

Adaptation

Most people's bodies will respond and adapt to the amount of physical demand placed upon them. Underused bodies will need time to adapt and then progress to higher levels of fitness in the exercise class. Older people may require longer to progress to a higher level of fitness. The rule should be:– *gradual progression* in the workload undertaken by each member of the class, until each new level is reached and there is improvement in physical ability. Within a few weeks the body learns to cope more efficiently and exercise becomes easier.

Exercise note:–
Increasing the exercise workload may mean:
1. Gradually increasing the repetition of an exercise.
2. Adjustment of the length of the lever – making the exercise harder.

Instructor's safety check

A sensible balance between adaptation and increased workload needs to be achieved in the exercise programme.

1. Avoid too much too soon. People need adequate rest between exercise sessions (three well spaced sessions per week).
2. Allow time in the exercise for muscles to contract and also allow a good stretch. Jerky fast movements may cause a reflex action which inhibits muscle flexibility and causes tension.
3. Avoid exercises which are inherently jerky or ballistic. Even the aerobic jog (which can cause tightening of the calf muscle) needs to be counterbalanced with complementary stretching exercise, e.g., hamstring stretches in the warm down period.
4. Body conditioning exercise which overloads the muscle, particularly those on the floor, need to be varied and interspersed with opportunities to relax the muscle to avoid 'burn', soreness and tightness from overuse.
5. Always provide the 'opt out' factor, offering people the chance to stop and rest. This will reduce any feeling of competition or failure to keep up among class members.

---

3. Changing the speed of the exercise – faster or slower
4. Changing the type of exercise.

Gravity

The movement produced by muscular contraction always works either in conjunction with or against gravity. Movement may be aided by gravity when it goes in the same direction, i.e., relaxing forward and down, or resist gravity when it pushes away, i.e., rising upward. The force of gravity may be neutralised in a sitting or standing at rest position. The centre of gravity in the body is said to be approximately at the level of the 2nd sacral vertebra.

Changing the position of the body will cause certain muscles to become more active. These muscles work against gravity to help stabilise and balance the body, and are large and powerful. They are found at the back of the hip, front of the thigh, and in the lower back and abdominal area.

Instructor's safety check

1. Successful execution of exercise movement depends on a class member's ability to direct and control the forces resulting from muscular contraction.

   Constant observation by the teacher is needed to spot misdirection of forces. Check:

   Correct positioning of the body
   Correct direction of movement to ensure use of chosen muscle groups and avoid stress.
   Correct involvement of all joints to ensure even distribution of force.

2. In choosing the exercises, try to sequence movements from larger muscle groups to smaller ones to ensure a smooth flowing progression.

3. Avoid too rapid acceleration of movement, combined with forceful muscle contraction (ballistic, bouncing movement). Forceful movement at high speed is unwise in a large group and will generally result in overstretched ligaments and muscle soreness and possibly stress to those joints involved.

Exercise note:–

Muscles that work against gravity work in pairs to support the body. Where there is a weaker development of one set of muscles the movement may be unbalanced, e.g., hip flexors and abdominal muscles work together; strong hip flexors and weak abdominal muscles will result in the pelvis rotating downward, producing lordosis (hollow back).

Balance or Equilibrium

The stability and balance of the body is affected by the force of gravity. Stability is achieved when body weight (centre of gravity) is aligned over its support base. The larger the base of support, the more stable the body. The lower the centre of gravity, the more stable the body.

Exercise note:

When we are thrown off balance, we quickly move other parts of the body to regain balance. This will involve a muscular reflex action.

Programme design

In planning the exercise programme gravity can be used to advantage. Exercises can be made more difficult by increasing the size of the body part which is being supported or lifted. Thus, a greater force is needed to maintain the body position or move it.

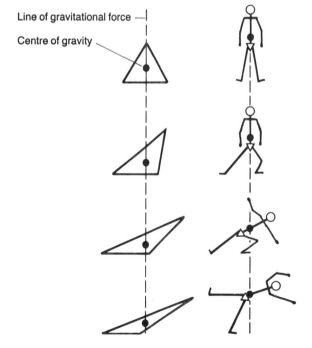

Line of gravitational force
Centre of gravity

Stable
Line of gravitational force well within base.

Less Stable
Line of gravitational force to one side of base.

Only Just Stable
Line of gravitational force almost outside base.

Unstable
Line of gravitational force well outside base.

Physiology

Physiology is the branch of medical science that deals with the healthy functions of different organs. A specific study of the physiology of exercise gives information about the changes that take place in the whole body in the course of its activities.

Exercise has an immediate effect upon bodily functions. In particular, exercise makes increased demands upon the various physiological systems which, over a period of time, improve their overall strength and efficiency and produce a feeling of fitness.

The focus of study in this section will be concerned with the structures which play a part in such physiological systems as the cardiovascular and respiratory functions of the body, (heart, circulation of blood, lungs), the production of energy and the relevance of the *aerobic* exercise programme toward the stimulation of increased levels of fitness.

The Cardiovascular System

The continuous process by which blood is pumped around the body to supply the cells and tissues with oxygen and nutrients, is a function of the *cardiovascular* system, which includes the heart and circulatory system.

The heart is a large muscle contained in a blood-filled bag, about the size of a fist, which operates as a pump circulating blood around the body. It is a hollow organ divided by a wall, or *septum* a left and right side. Each side is then divided again into a smaller upper section, the *atrium,* and a larger lower section, the *ventricle.*

The *cardiac muscle* of the heart contracts about 70 times a minute (at rest) to pump blood around the body, in a continuous

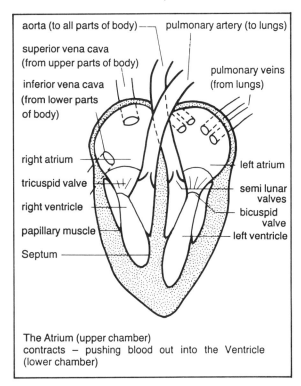

aorta (to all parts of body) — pulmonary artery (to lungs)

superior vena cava (from upper parts of body)

pulmonary veins (from lungs)

inferior vena cava (from lower parts of body)

right atrium

left atrium

tricuspid valve

semi lunar valves

right ventricle

bicuspid valve

papillary muscle

left ventricle

Septum

The Atrium (upper chamber) contracts – pushing blood out into the Ventricle (lower chamber)

rhythm of contraction and relaxation. The period of contraction is known as *systole,* while the period of relaxation is called *diastole.* A cardiac centre in the brain stem controls the rate and strength of the contractions as required by changing demands made upon the body.

The heart is really two pumps. The pump on the right side receives blood as it returns from the body and pumps it through the lungs to be purified and collect oxygen. The pump on the left side receives the blood, which has been oxygenated, from the lungs and pumps it out to all parts of the body.

The Circulatory System

The circulatory system is a large network of piping whose function is to transport the blood around the body. It consists of *arteries* and *veins,* which divide into smaller *arterioles* and *venules,* then further divide into tiny *capillaries* within the tissue.

Arteries. With the exception of the pulmonary artery, arteries carry oxygenated and nutrient-rich blood from the heart to the tissues. Blood leaves the heart via the aorta which is the largest artery in the body. Arterial walls are tough, thick and elastic to withstand the high pressure of blood flowing through them. The power of the ventricular contraction of the heart, together with the elasticity of the artery wall, ensures the forward flow of arterial blood. With increasing distance from the heart, arteries become smaller, branching into arterioles, and finally into networks of capillaries in the tissues. The walls of the smaller arteries and arterioles contain more muscle tissue to allow them to be more adaptable, to dilate and contract according to the needs of the body, thus regulating the flow of blood. The heart receives its own blood supply via the *coronary arteries.*

Exercise note:
Over a period of time, sometimes starting in early life, the walls of the arteries can gradually become furred up with fatty deposits called atheroma. This substance can become too thick, causing a narrowing in the arteries. Where this occurs in a coronary artery the blood supply to the heart muscle may be restricted or even blocked. This is *coronary heart disease.* When increased activity places demands upon the body, making the heart pump faster, this starvation of blood to the heart, due to restricted flow causes excruciating pain known as *angina.*

When blood cannot get through to a part of the heart muscle because of a blockage (blood clot) – *coronary thrombosis* – it does not receive oxygen. This may cause the heart to stop pumping altogether resulting in a heart attack – *cardiac arrest.*

Heart disease is silent and insidious, and the warnings of its presence may not always be observed. Prevention is better than cure.
MOTTO: Make regular exercise a part of a healthy lifestyle.

Capillaries are extremely fine vessels forming networks in the tissues. Those that branch from arterioles are responsible for the exchange of oxygen and other nutrients with the cells of the body, via their thin walls. Capillaries that branch from venules carry away waste products and carbon dioxide from the cells. It is from the capillaries that the venous return to the heart begins.

Veins. The waste products collected from the cells by the capillaries are conveyed into the venules which then merge to form the larger veins, whose function is to carry deoxygenated blood back to the heart. Veins have thinner less elastic walls than arteries and so exert less pressure to push the blood back to the heart. However, their walls contain one-way valves which prevent a back flow of blood into the capillaries. In the limbs, where blood travels against gravity, these valves are situated at irregular intervals along the vein wall, allowing the blood to be caught and held and helped to move forward. The surrounding muscles also provide a stimulating action on the vein wall to help push the blood along.

Heart Rate, Pulse and Blood Pressure

When blood is pumped out of the heart, a wave of increased pressure is felt in the arteries. This *arterial pulse* can best be felt where the artery crosses a bone and lies superficially, i.e., at the front of the wrist, throat or temple.

The pumping rate of the heart is governed by varying factors:

> age
> degree of fitness
> lifestyle/working environment/
> sedentary nature of work and leisure activity/stress factors/diet/body weight/ alcohol consumption/smoking.

The normal resting pulse rate for an adult is between 60 and 80 beats per minute. This will increase during exercise.

Cardiac output is the amount of blood that can be circulated by the heart to the body per minute. This is calculated by multiplying the stroke (volume of blood pumped out by one contraction of left ventricle) by the heart rate (beats per minute.)

Therefore, cardiac output = stroke volume (SV) x beats per minutes (BPM).

In a normal, resting adult, cardiac output = 70ml (SV) x 75 (BPM) = 5.25 litres blood pumped round the body per minute.

Exercise note:

1. During exercise the heart and pulse rate is increased, as is the volume of blood leaving the heart. The circulation of blood is redistributed to the heart muscles and skeletal muscles.
2. Vessels in the skin dilate to allow heat regulation.
3. Vessels in the digestive tract will close temporarily.

Blood pressure is the pressure applied by the heart and arteries to propel the blood around the body. The left ventricle forces blood into the *aorta* and the pressure rises to a peak – *systiolic pressure.* As the ventricle empties of blood the pressure then falls during *diastole* (resting state). If the diastolic pressure is too high, i.e., over 100 mm Hg, then the heart is having to work under too much pressure and a potentially harmful state of high blood pressure, or *hypertension,* exists.

Blood pressure depends partly upon the stroke volume of the blood pumped from the heart to the body and partly on the contraction of the muscles in the artery walls; the latter is governed by a centre (the medulla oblongata) in the brain stem.

Exercise note:

A person may not always realise they have high blood pressure as he may feel normal.

Nevertheless, the overworking of the heart and the 'furring' of the arteries can lead to the danger of a heart attack.

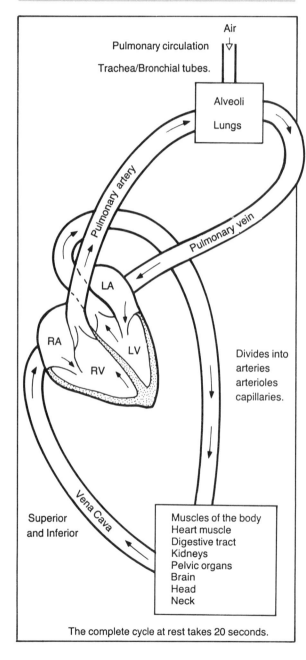

The complete cycle at rest takes 20 seconds.

The Oxygen Transport System

In order for the body to function, a constant supply of oxygen is needed by the tissues. Muscles cannot work without oxygen. The provision of oxygen to the muscle cell is dependent upon the body coordinating the activities of the cardiovascular system with the respiratory system, i.e., lungs. The cardiovascular respiratory function of the body requires an efficient oxygen transport system.

Pulmonary circulation: The cycle of blood through the lungs. In the heart the right ventricle (RV) pumps deoxygenated blood up the pulmonary artery to the lungs, where carbon dioxide is exchanged for oxygen. Oxygenated blood then returns, via the pulmonary vein, to the left atrium (LA) of the heart.

Systemic circulation: The cycle of blood round the body and back to the heart. The left ventricle (LV) of the heart pumps oxygenated blood, i.e., arterial blood, via the aorta, to all parts of the body. Deoxygenated blood, i.e., venous blood, returns from the tissues via the superior and inferior vena cava, to the right atrium (RA) of the heart. The complete cycle, at rest, takes about 20 seconds.

Oxygen Transport System during Exercise:

At the onset of exercise the rate and depth of respiration increases as the demand for oxygen in the lungs is stepped up.

Air moves down the trachea (windpipe) into the bronchial tubes of the lungs.

In the many tiny alveoli of the lungs, more capillaries open up to allow for exchange of carbon dioxide for oxygen over a greater surface area than at rest.

More of the oxygen-carrying pigment (haemoglobin) in the red blood cells combines with the greater supply of oxygen molecules.

More oxygenated blood is then carried through the pulmonary veins to the heart, causing greater expansion of the left atrium.

More oxygenated blood is pumped by the left ventricle at each beat (stroke volume) and the heart rate increases. As a result a greater volume of blood is pumped from the heart, through the aorta, round the body each minute (i.e., cardiac output is increased).

Blood is diverted to the areas of high activity especially muscles, where demand for oxygen and nutrients is greatest. Here, *aerobic metabolism* takes place (glycogen is broken down in the presence of oxygen to produce energy, see p.32), and the rate of metabolic activity is increased in relation to the demand for energy.

Larger amounts of carbon dioxide and water are produced as waste products of metabolism and are carried away by the blood.

A greater volume of deoxygenated blood is carried back to the right atrium of the heart through the veins.

More deoxygenated blood is pumped through (the pulmonary arteries from the right ventricle of the heart in order to eliminate the greater levels of carbon dioxide and to establish the balance with the new intake of oxygen to the lungs.

Energy Production

We can liken the body to a machine in its structure and function, with the heart as the motor from which the life support systems radiate on their arterial network of connecting pathways. Also like a machine, the body requires fuel to power the system. This supply of fuel is needed constantly in order to produce *energy* to keep the body functioning.

Energy is essential for each of us to pursue our daily tasks with vigour, both in work and leisure time. The fuel which the body requires comes from three sources:

1. Oxygen from the lungs.
2. Carbohydrates (sugars and starches) digested from food we eat and then stored in the liver and muscles.
3. Fat, derived from our food and stored all over the body.

In the cells the carbohydrates and fats are broken down during *metabolism,* through a chemical reaction involving oxygen, to yield a compound called *adenosine triphosphate,* or ATP, which functions as a carrier of energy. When ATP is itself broken down, a large amount of energy is released for immediate use by the muscles.

Muscular energy comes from three types of metabolic systems: creatine phosphate, anaerobic (lactic acid) system, and aerobic (oxygen) system.

Creatine Phosphate (CP) System. A limited supply of energy is present in the muscle for immediate use, in the form of creatine phosphate (CP) which is a source of ATP. This supply is only temporary and sufficient only for a short burst of activity.

Exercise Note:
At rest only a small amount of energy is needed, some of which will come from CP metabolism. At the onset of exercise there will be a sudden requirement for more energy, and this will place a greater demand on the sources of stored energy. The CP system will only meet this demand for the first 30 seconds of exercise, after which it is depleted.

Anaerobic (Lactic Acid) System. Anaerobic metabolism takes over when exercise intensifies. It provides a fast supply of energy, produced by the breakdown of the carbohydrate *glycogen* which is stored in the liver and muscles. This process of conversion which does not involve oxygen produces *lactic acid* as a by-product, which accumulates largely in the blood and muscles.

Exercise Note:

Anaerobic training requires short periods (1-3 minutes) of strenuous activity, followed by inactivity and periods of rest. Anaerobic exercise quickly uses up the glycogen stored in the muscles. If there is a build up of lactic acid in the muscles and blood, fatigue will result.

Aerobic (oxygen) system. Where exercise activity is continuous, the body relies mostly upon the aerobic system of metabolism for its supply of energy (as it does at rest). The fuel for this is provided by fat, glycogen and oxygen. The chemical reaction of fat or glycogen with oxygen produces ATP, together with carbon dioxide and water as waste products. Aerobic metabolism can cope adequately in meeting the body's demands for a supply of energy if the demands are not excessive.

Exercise Note:

In aerobic training, the ability is developed to breathe in large volumes of air, and to circulate its oxygen effectively through the lungs and heart into the body and throughout the muscular system, for energy production.

The continuous nature of aerobic exercise builds up the endurance and strength of heart and lungs, improving overall physical fitness.

The more oxygen one can supply to the muscles, the longer they will be able to keep working and the less quickly they will tire.

Aerobic Principles (FITT)

The most relevant test of a person's fitness is the *aerobic capacity*. This is a measurement of one's ability to take up oxygen, transport it efficiently through the bloodstream and produce energy within the muscles.

Aerobic capacity is the single most important indicator of physical fitness. The more oxygen one can supply to the muscles, the more efficiently they will be able to contract and so the greater will be the capacity for exercise, and the longer the muscles will take to tire.

Aerobic capacity will improve through sustained heart and lung activity brought about by exercise of sufficient *frequency (F), intensity (I) duration of time (T)*, and of a particular *type (T)*, to challenge the cardiovascular respiratory functions of the body and bring about a training effect.

Frequency of Exercise

Frequency refers to the number of exercise sessions taken per week. It is generally considered that three times is the minimum amount required to improve and maintain a fitness level, bearing in mind that, other than dance exercise, other forms of aerobic exercise may be taken, for example cycling / swimming / skipping / brisk walking / jogging / circuit training.

Intensity of Exercise

Since during exercise the heart rate increases in proportion to the intensity of the activity, this is used as a monitor of the individual's raised level of physical stress. This measure gives an indication of:

1. A class member's progress over time.

2. Guidelines for maintaining safety levels of exercise activity.

The heart rate is measured by taking the pulse, either at the wrist (radial pulse) or at the throat (carotid pulse).

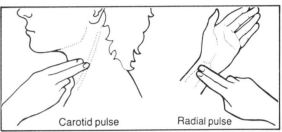

Carotid pulse   Radial pulse

In order to calculate the heart rate per minute which represents a safe level for the individual, you need first to be aware of the normal resting heart rate. This should be between 60 and 90 beats per minute, although some people may have a rate naturally lower or higher than this. To obtain a more accurate calculation of the true resting heart rate, it is good practice to take the pulse on waking, for 15 seconds, then multiply by 4 to find the rate per minute.

Once the body starts to respond aerobically to the increased intensity of the exercise session, greater demands are placed on the heart's working capacity and the heart rate rises. In order to monitor the safety levels for each individual you need to be aware of the maximum attainable heart rate (MHR) for that person's age group, which is obtained by a simple calculation:

Women MHR = 220 – Age
e.g., the MHR for a 40-year old woman is:
220 – 40 = 180 beats per minute

Men MHR = 205 – Half age
e.g., the MHR for a 40-year old man is:
205 – 20 = 185 beats per minute

In fact, a beat is lost for each year of your life.

In order to achieve a training effect every person needs to work at a percentage of this maximum level. This personal training heart rate can be based at an appropriate level to suit their own needs, for example, 60 per cent for a beginner, 70 per cent for intermediate, and 90 per cent for advanced. The training heart rate (THR) is found by multiplying the maximum heart rate by the percentage required:

MHR × % = THR
e.g., THR for a 40-year old woman at 70 per cent of maximum is:
180 × 70/100 = 126 beats per minute

Target Zone for Heart Rate

Since it is difficult for class members to make arithmetical calculations, especially after the concentration required by the more demanding aerobic session, it is a good idea to have on display a large chart which sets out different age groups and indicates minimum and maximum percentage heart rates, thus giving a heart rate target zone within which to work. This visual aid will simplify matters for the class and the instructor, and will give an instant easy reference of safety levels and also of week by week improvement in fitness. The percentage heart rate can be adjusted as fitness improvement takes place.

The information could also be presented to provide immediate reference, as follows:

Age	Predicted maximum heart rate (beats/minute)	60% (beginners)	70% (intermediate)	90% (advanced)
20	200	120	140	180
25	195	117	136	176
30	190	114	133	171
35	185	111	130	167
40	180	108	126	163
45	175	105	123	159
50	170	102	119	154
55	165	99	116	150
60	160	96	112	146

Exercise note:
It is probable that, within the average exercise class, there will be people of all ages, levels of fitness and with varying degrees of skill in physical agility.

It may be useful to encourage a self-awareness among class members by helping them to monitor certain signals from their own bodies:

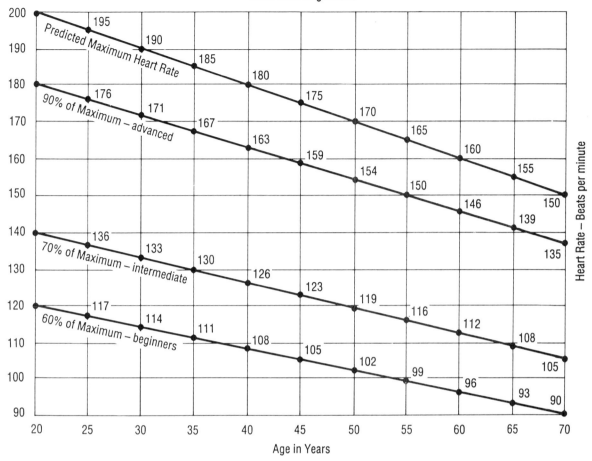

Heart Rate Target Zone

1. *Breathing* should be harder than at rest but not gasping for breath.
   Test: Can you talk to your neighbour after the aerobic session?
   Does normal breathing return within 5 minutes of warm down?

2. *Dizzyness.* This is not normal if the aerobic activity has been carried out at an appropriate level. Advise walking down activity and avoid any exercise which takes the head down to floor level.

3. *Stitch or cramps.* These are conditions of a lack of circulation to the muscle. Advise walking down or working at a lower level while remembering to breathe, until normality is resumed.

4. *Pain.* In the chest may be an indication of excessive exercise affecting the flow of blood to the heart. Have this checked medically.

   Pain. In a limb or joint may be an indication of an improper alignment of the body during exercise, causing twisting or tearing of the ligament, or a too vigorous, ballistic approach to the movement. Lessen the intensity of the exercise and check posture.

5. *Excessive fatigue.* Exercising aerobically should produce energy. Stamina needs to build slowly over time. Work at a comfortable level at first, until higher levels can be achieved.

Time (Duration) of Exercise

Time and intensity tend to be inter related qualities of exercise activity. A short period, e.g., 10 minutes of high level, strenuous activity will produce an anaerobic response but may also be distressing or uncomfortable. A longer period, e.g., 15 to 20 minutes, of moderate intensity activity will raise the heart rate within the target zone and achieve a training effect, while minimising fatigue and discomfort.

The latter is a safer and more efficient level at which to aim class activity for the average individual, bearing in mind that time will have been allowed for the preceding warm up and for the warm down session to follow.

Type of Exercise

The type of exercise activity chosen for the aerobic section of the programme will largely depend on the instructor's background in movement training and individual preference. In general, the exercise activity should be composed of calisthenics, involving the large muscle groups, and a variety of stepping, hopping, travelling, skipping movements. Depending on the instructor's skills, there is scope for the introduction of a large variety of simple dance steps.

Instructor's safety check

1. As a general rule: the larger the steps and arm movements, the greater the force required to execute the activity and the higher the heart rate. Smaller steps and arm movements require less force and produce a lower heart rate.

There is therefore scope for increasing the intensity of exercise for individuals who wish to work harder, or for lowering the intensity for those who wish to sustain a moderate approach, through varying the type of exercise performed.

Programme Design

It is necessary for the instructor to plan the exercise activity at a 'middle of the road' level, particularly where class members vary from week to week and new members are constantly arriving. However, there is need for a 'step down' option at a lower level for beginners, and a 'step up' option to challenge the more advanced members of the class.

NB It is entirely up to the instructor to indicate all three levels, week by week, reminding class members to work at their own individual levels, thus eliminating any competitive atmosphere or fear of failure to keep up.

Safety Considerations

The goal of every class instructor should be to conduct a safe class in a safe environment. The responsibility for these aspects of safety lies totally with the instructor.

Aerobic exercise is not an easy way to get fit. For the unfit, overweight candidate it will be hazardous to participate fully in high level exercise activity straight away. Injuries can arise from too much, too soon. It is best to build up slowly through a sensibly graded programme of exercise, allowing the body's tolerance of exercise to increase gradually.

This section is concerned with an understanding of the dangers associated with exercise, preventative measures to take to guard against possible injuries (fitness class precautions), and reference for elementary first aid skills to deal with emergency situation. Vulnerable areas of the body are also discussed, together with exercises which may be potentially harmful.

General Precautions in the Exercise Class

An exercise class is composed of individuals who will vary in age, level of fitness, physical ability and medical history. Because exercise places the body under a form of physical stress, it is necessary for the instructor to be aware of the class as individuals, and to gain the necessary information through a screening process. This will classify class members according to their level of fitness, or any risks which may be involved, so indicating their eligibility for participation in the exercise programme.

Health and Fitness Screening

Screening can be used to evaluate a person's current level of fitness and physical state, which should give an indication of their suitability to begin an exercise programme and eliminate any risk factors. The screening process should include questions about a class member's medical history and general lifestyle.

Several types of health and fitness screening are available through both the private and public health sectors. Many of the larger health clubs offer basic assessments of fitness as part of their service, while at a more sophisticated level, full medical tests are available from the private health clinics, many of which are being established nationwide. Information concerning the availability of such tests can be made available to the class if the instructor first does some research in the locality.

An estimation of individual health and fitness can be obtained at class level if some guidelines are observed, involving fore-knowledge of fitness level and risk factors appertaining to each class member.

Screening at Class Level

1. *Information*. Keep a filing system, logging:
   names and addresses,
   Age
   Resting heart rate
   Target heart rate zone
   Any medical information which may appear contraindicative to some types of exercise.

2. *Risk factors*. By using large posters around the room, draw attention to risk factors, for example:
   Have your recently had an operation?
   Are you pregnant?
   Have you recently had a baby?
   Are you currently receiving medical treatment?
   Are you overweight?
   Do you suffer from pain in any joint?
   Are you aged over 35 years and unused to exercise?

3. *Questionnaire*. Provide a large questionnaire, prominently displayed alongside your target heart rate zone chart, which asks the following questions.

   Do you suffer from:

Diabetes	Yes/No
High blood pressure	Yes/No
Joint or back pain problems	Yes/No
Headaches	Yes/No
Overweight	Yes/No
Dizziness/fainting	Yes/No

Have you recently:

Had a baby	Yes/No
Had an operation	Yes/No
Received medical treatment	Yes/No
Suffered chest pains after exertion	Yes/No

Are you aged over 35 years and unused to exercise?

Make sure that every class member has been talked through the questionnaire on a one-to-one basis, in a relaxed manner, and fully understands the implications of embarking on the exercise programme.

Instructor's safety check

1. Pre-screen to classify class members according to medical background and lifestyle, to provide a starting point for the class instructor to become acquainted with members.

2. Monitor pulse rates on a regular basis and record

3. Educate class members to be aware of personal limitations, to avoid overexertion, and to work at a level for them.

4. Advise a medical check up if the answer is YES to any of the questions on the questionnaire.

5. Discourage the competitive element.

Class Environment
Consideration needs to be given to the facilities which are provided and the general environment within which the class is conducted. When looking for a suitable location for the class, several safety factors should influence your choice.

Space. Equate the amount of space available with the projected size of your class. A small, cramped room with internal obstructions (pillars, chairs, tables, etc.) will restrict the number of people who can safely move around.

Temperature. Be conversant with the type of heating and ventilation used. The room needs to be comfortably warm at the onset of exercise, particularly in Winter, and well ventilated to prevent lack of oxygen, especially after the aerobic section, or in hot weather. Access to a drink of water will be appreciated.

Floor surface. Ideally, the floor should be clean, smooth and well sprung to give extra resilience to the body during exercise activity. Failing this a wooden floor is preferable to any other kind. Avoid concrete or carpet-covered concrete as such surfaces will only produce a jarring effect on the joints during any kind of jumping or jogging exercise. The composition-type floor generally found in sports centres is not ideal.

Correct clothing and footwear. Clothing should be comfortable and appropriate to movement activity, e.g., leotard, tights, track suit. Loose layers are preferable to garments that are too tight. Leg warmers and sweat shirts are not just 'trendy' garments, but help keep muscles warm at the beginning of exercise. They can be removed as the body heats up and put on again for the cool down period.

The instructor can advise her class members on pointers to look for when buying an aerobic dance shoe. The shoe should be:

1. Lightweight and supportive, designed specifically for aerobic dance exercise. Not a track shoe for running.

2. Flexible to assist the range of movement required in footwork activity.

3. Shock absorbent and cushioned, designed to dissipate the shock effect of the foot striking the floor.

4. Well fitting, allowing room for the feet to swell slightly during exercise, preventing blisters. Avoid the shoe with a high back tab, which puts pressure on the Achilles tendon.

5. In very hot conditions advise wearing a natural fibre sock to absorb perspiration.

Instructor's safety check

Encourage class members to wear appropriate clothing and footwear.

Footwear. Shoes are preventive equipment for the feet because they act as shock absorbers. The stress produced from jogging, skipping or running activity increases the body weight, which is largely felt and absorbed by the ankles, knees and lower back. It is very important to avoid injury by wearing correct shoes during the aerobic class.

Making sure that your class members are comfortable and protected in their environment helps to promote you as a caring instructor.

Vulnerable Body Areas

The human body is very adaptable and can, with training and practice, achieve a remarkable range and facility of movement. It can even cope with exercise movements which are generally considered harmful. The risks of this practice, however, may far outweigh the benefits. The instructor should be well acquainted with the most common injury sites in aerobic dance exercise and dance-related exercise, and avoid the incidence of injuries which fall into the 'overuse' category, caused by the overload which occurs in endurance exercise. Selecting the appropriate content of an exercise programme is dealt with more fully in Section 5 (p. 54).

Areas particularly prone to damage are the ankle, neck, lower back and other spinal structures, and the knee. Knowledge of the anatomy and relevant biomechanics related to these areas can lead to a better understanding of the causes of injury and therefore of how to prevent its occurrence.

The Ankle

The ankle region is a centre for many functions:–

1. It is capable of producing power to elevate the body.

2. It acts as a shock absorber to prevent jarring and stress to other parts of the body in running and jumping activities.

3. It is a receptor area for the body's sense of balance.

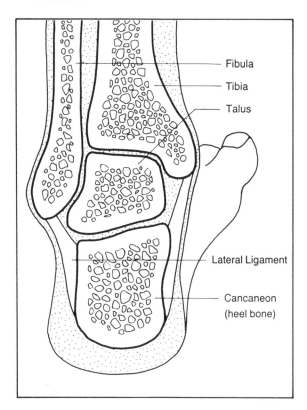

Fibula
Tibia
Talus
Lateral Ligament
Cancaneon
(heel bone)

The bones of the ankle fit together within a strong capsule, to which they are attached. The capsule is further strengthened by an outer and inner ligament which prevent the ankle from any excessive movement.

The ligaments tend to be inelastic, and the outer ligament is weaker than the inner.

Exercise note:
Movements such as running, jumping and skipping can result in awkward landing, twisting the ankle, and causing a lateral ligament sprain on the outside of the joint.

Alternatively, an overbalance can cause the foot to twist inwards under the full body weight, causing an inversion sprain. This occurs because of the greater freedom of movement inward and the weakness of the lateral ligament, which can easily be overstretched.

Overuse tendonitis, particularly Achilles tendonitis, which occurs in the Achilles tendon, is a very painful overuse injury. The tendon becomes inflamed at its insertion on the bone and the whole area becomes tender and sore, with recovery taking as much as three weeks complete rest.

Instructor's safety check

Overuse injuries may occur unnoticed from constant misuse of feet and ankles during exercise, placing a minor repetitive stress over time.

1. Ankle strengthening exercises should be included in your programme.
    e.g., Plantarflexion
    Dorsiflexion
    Inversion and eversion stretches
    Rotation

2. Avoid rolling or bouncing on the ankles.

3. Where rising or balancing, keep the foot square, not rolling in or out. Particularly in jogging activity, maintain good alignment and don't allow the ankle to take the strain.

The Neck and Lower Back

The same principles as apply to the ankle also apply to the neck (cervical spine) and the lower back (lumbar spine), when considering their vulnerability to damage.

The human spine undergoes various changes in posture in its development from foetus to adult.

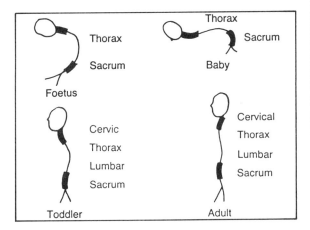

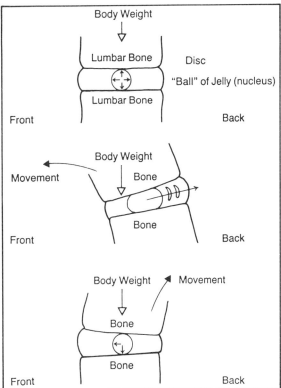

The thorax and sacrum (tailbone) remain as primary curves, or curves into forward flexion, throughout life, and this thoracic and sacral curvature is present at birth.

The cervical and lumbar curvatures develop as the child matures and alter to *secondary curves,* or curves into *extension.* It is this change, together with their flexibility, which predisposes and makes them prone to injury.

Spinal Structures

The vertebrae of the spine are separated by intervertebral discs and linked to facet joints and arches, all stacked on top of each other, bound by ligaments and supported by muscles.

When we look at the disc between the bones, we can see which movements are likely to induce an injury, which structures are injured and why there is a high level of associated pain.

At rest, the body weight should fall through the centre of the disc, through its soft 'ball bearing', or nucleus.

In forward flexion, the back of the disc is stretched. The body weight falls in front of the nucleus, compressing the disc, forcing the nucleus back and weakening the ring of tough disc around it. Therefore, the delicate structures (nerves and ligaments) behind the disc are at risk of injury.

In extension, however, the converse applies. The disc is kept central or forwards, with little or no compression. It is therefore ESSENTIAL to preserve the secondary curve of the lumbar spine if it is loaded with body weight, as in sitting or standing. At the least, if you have to flex forwards, compensate by leaning backwards (extending) afterwards.

The back of the disc is very close to many delicate structures, not least the spinal cord! If we look slightly to the side of the spinal cord we can see the various neurological structures more usually compressed by a prolapsed disc.

41

Any pressure on the spinal nerves in this region may cause intense pain.

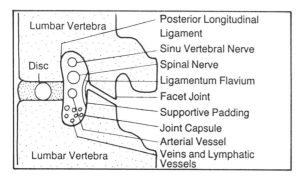

Lumbar Vertebra — Posterior Longitudinal Ligament
— Sinu Vertebral Nerve
Disc — Spinal Nerve
— Ligamentum Flavium
— Facet Joint
— Supportive Padding
— Joint Capsule
— Arterial Vessel
Lumbar Vertebra — Veins and Lymphatic Vessels

If the secondary curve is lost and the lower back is perpetually flexed, injury and pain will result. Any imbalance in strength between the abdominal muscles and the spinal muscles will produce an incorrect or flexed posture of the lumbar spine, and therefore a tendency to injury.

Consider the load in lbs of pressure recorded inside the disc in various positions.

1. Lying flat, supine   30
2. Sitting unsupported   100
3. Standing correctly   80–85
4. Standing with 20 degrees of flexion   120
5. Standing with 20 degrees of flexion holding 10 Kg in each hand   185
6. Lifting 40 Kg correctly (knees bent, back straight)   180–210
7. Lifting 40 Kg badly (knees straight, back bent)   310
8. Sit-up exercise (straight legs)   210
9. Sit-up exercise (bent legs)   180
10. Active extension lying prone (on stomach)   150
11. Static abdominal exercises   110

Exercise note:
Repeated toe-touching with a curved back, or vigorous combined movements with rotation and flexion for both the lower back and neck, are injury inducing.

Instructor's safety check

The intervertebral discs are thicker in the cervical and lumbar regions and thinner in the thoracic region of the spine. This means that the spine enjoys a greater freedom of movement in the former areas and consequently a possibly greater susceptibility to injury there.

Neck
1. Avoid all circular head movements. The weight of the head (22-26.5 Kg or 10-12 lbs) acted on by gravity, plus tight muscles, brings the vertebrae closer together and can grind them.

2. Keep head movements slow and controlled – never violent and jerky or floppy.

3. Be cautious when the head is held back, as this shortens and tightens the muscles at the back of the neck and needs a compensatory release.

   NB this situation can occur in some held-back positions at floor level where the class is observing the teacher.

4. Always think 'long back', pulling up from the top of the head, chin parallel to floor.

Low back
1. Avoid hyperextension (arching) of the back, as this puts a great deal of pressure on joints and can cause pain.

2. Encourage the pelvic tilt exercise either standing or lying. This forward rotation of the pelvis decreases the arch in the lower back and relieves pressure on the joints.

3. Standing side stretches (lateral flexion) need checking for alignment. Think of body between two boards, tucking the hips under so that abdomen can support the lower back.

NB Flat back – Forward flexion of the spine standing.

This tends to come into the grey zone category of controversial exercises. Where it may be an appropriate exercise for, say, 'a group of trained dancers', it may not be for 'the average housewife'. If the Flat Back is to be attempted, move into it in a controlled manner and check alignment, i.e., hips over feet, tummy up, long spine (no dips or bumps). Remember neck and head are part of the spine, pulling forward looking at floor and keeping the knees slightly relaxed rather than locked out. Arms may rest on thighs or extend at side rather than forward, which adds weight and length to the leverage and thus increases stress in the lower back. Always recover from the Flat Back position through a curled spine and bent knees.

BUT – WHEN IN DOUBT, LEAVE IT OUT!

The Knee

The knee is a complex hinge joint with many articular peculiarities. For example, unlike a simple hinge joint, it allows some rotation of the shin bone (tibia) upon the thigh bone (femur). The knee cap (patella) also articulates with the front of the thigh bone.

The knee is heavily prone to injury because:
a) it is a weight-bearing joint
b) it has many periarticular and intra-articular structures easily damaged by overuse and misuse.

The long bones, such as the tibia, cease to grow at about 18-20 years of age when the epiphysis or growing plate fuses with the main shaft of the bone. Exercise activity in children, which involves too much pounding or jarring movement may permanently damage the knee joint, so it is inadvisable for them to participate in high level aerobic jogging. Consider that the compression force at the upper tibial epiphysis is 1½ times body weight when walking, and 7 times body weight when running or jumping. Therefore, even in adult participation in aerobic jogging, care must be taken to ensure that the floor is suitable (preferably wooden and sprung), and that footwear is cushioned and supportive, to avoid concussive injury. The knee is happiest and at its most stable point when in full extension, and when the ligaments at the side are tight.

The knee is at its most vulnerable and unstable point when semiflexed, weight bearing and with a twist or lean. Where the knee joint is continuously subjected to too much compression with full weight bearing and added rotary component (as in squat thrusts) injuries such as bucket-handled tears of the cartilage, torn menisci, inflamed bursae, and torn muscle and ligament can all result.

The knee joint itself has the following structures in and around it:

1. Two half-moon cartilages, one each side of the central ridges of the tibial surface.
2. Two cruciate ligaments, so called because they form a cross, which help hold the femur and tibia in close alignment.
3. A transverse ligament running from edge to edge of the cartilages at the front.
4. An inside edge or medial ligament across the joint.
5. An outside edge or lateral ligament.
6. The 'arcuate popliteal ligament' at the back.
7. A joint capsule.
8. Several cushioning fluid sacs called bursae – four at the front, four at the outside, and five on the inside.
9. A fatty pad under the patella, extending into the joint.
10. Tough supporting sheets, called 'retinacula', on either side of the patella.
11. Tendons of 12 muscles.
12. Nerves.
13. Blood vessels and lymph nodes and vessels.

In other words, plenty to injure!

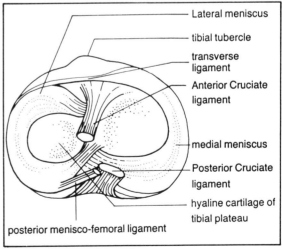

Tibial component of (L) knee joint viewed from above, demonstrating tibial attachments of the cruciate ligaments and the medial and lateral menisci.

Controversial Exercises

It is true to say that any exercise can be damaging if it is badly executed. Unfortunately, with the best will in the world, a movement executed well by the teacher may be poorly interpreted by a class member through poor posture, bad alignment or lack of body control. This will result in stress or damage to the body. Given that the exercise class is not intended as a work out for the teacher, and that every attempt will be made to teach the exercise thoroughly and carefully throughout the class, there will probably still be some exercises which fall into a 'grey' area and cannot be positively identified as 'safe' or 'unsafe'.

A good way of deciding whether to include this type of exercise in your programme is first to assess the individuals within the group. What is good for a young, fit, athletic group will not be suitable for older, more mature class members. Within the group there may be people with a poor medical history who could present problems. How long has the group been exercising with you? What is its general technical ability, body control, flexibility, cardiovascular fitness, stamina, etc.

If you still wish to include a particular exercise, consider whether the benefits outweigh the risks. What are the benefits of the exercise? Try it out yourself to find the effect on muscle groups. What are the risks? What pressures and strains does it put on the body? Which parts of the body are likely to be affected? Finally if you decide to try out the exercise with your group – *always* point out the dangerous pressures exerted at specific points of the body and coach the correct body procedure. Afterwards, check out the exercise with the class and ask for feedback on how they felt performing it.

Contraindicated Exercises

The exercises listed under 'Don't' in the following table are now considered wholly unsuitable for anyone. Their original value or purpose has been outweighed by the risks involved to the body in their execution. Some safe alternatives are given ('do').

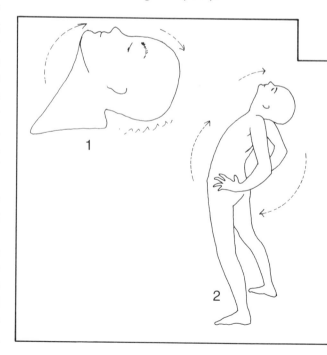

Contraindicated Exercises and Safe Alternatives

Fig. No.	Don't	Pressure Point	Do
1	Full rotation of the head, circling backward.	Neck Hyperextension of cervical spine, shortens and tightens muscles at back of neck. Can grind the bones.	Turning movements lateral flexion forward flexion, half-circle rotation forward.
2	Full rotation of the upper body, circling backward.	Back Hyperextension of lumbar spine, overarching, putting pressure on joints in lower back.	Lateral flexion half-turn sideways half-circle forward.
3	Flat Back Extreme forward flexion with added leverage and weight in arms.	Back Lumbar spine under pressure from extreme flexion, and over-stretching. Knee Knee joint locked. Hamstrings stretched tight.	Flat back with knees bent. Arms wide or hands on thighs. Touch toes in sitting position, one knee bent.
4	The Plough (Yoga)	Neck Places extreme pressure on the cervical spine.	Keep one knee bent to chest and slowly extend other leg within personal range of movement.
5	Straight leg sit-up	Back Hyperextension of lower back. Iliopsoas or hip flexor muscles take over, causing pelvis to rotate forwards lower back to come off floor.	Keep knees bent. Curl up to touch top of knees. Tilt the pelvis.
6	Straight leg raises.	Extreme overuse injuries here, would cause the anterior longitudinal ligament to strip off the front of the spine.	One knee bent, raise other leg.

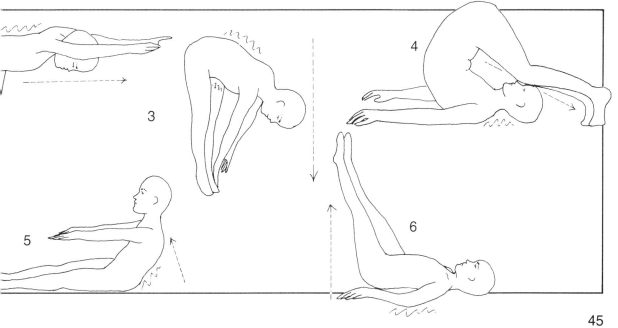

Fig. No.	Don't	Pressure Point	Do
1	Full knee bend or squat thrust.	Knee Cruciate ligaments of knee overstretched. Back Hyperextension of lower back.	Half bend knees to lower body to floor. Extend each leg back in turn, with control.
2	High leg kick back and up, from kneeling.	Back Hyperextension of lower back at full lift and extension of leg.	Rest weight lower on forearms. Lift one leg slowly with control and not too high. Kneel and lower and lift leg only to horizontal
3	Cobra stretch (Yoga)	Back Hyperextension of lower back.	Moderate the stretch. Hips on floor, arms bent.
4	Half rotation of upper torso — arms high.	Back Allows hips to move. Hyperextension in lower back. Knee ligaments twist.	Relax knees slightly. Lower arms. Hips square.

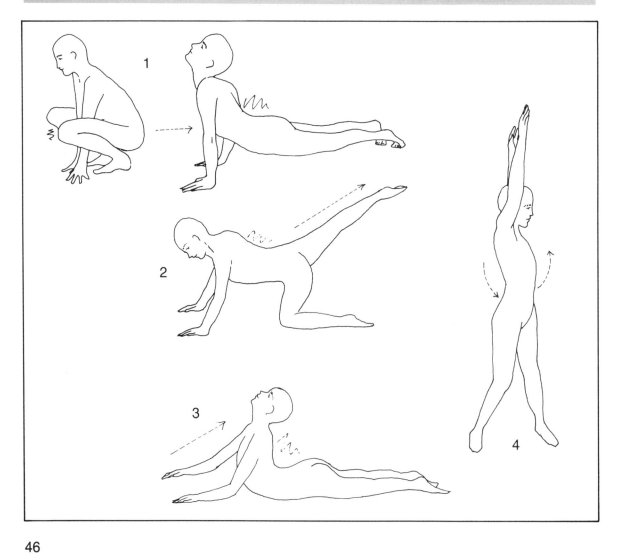

First Aid

The expertise required by the class instructor in the First Aid department falls into two categories. At the least he/she will be expected to adopt the role of clinical consultant, diagnosing the causes of many aches and pains and proffering advice on their treatment. At the most he/she will be expected to be knowledgeably equipped to deal with any unforeseen emergencies which may arise in the exercise class.

Minor Injuries and Discomforts

Some minor injuries that may occur and their treatment, are out-lined in the table.

Acute Injuries – Emergency Procedure

Whatever the apparent severity of the injury, it is the instructor's responsibility to act immediately, in as calm and controlled a manner as possible. He/she must deal with the emergency situation in such a way as to ensure the safety and well-being of the injured person, and to convey an air of confidence and responsibility to the remainder of the class.

Problem	Cause	Cure	Prevention
Faintness and sickness. Fatigue.	Lack of blood to brain, because it is being directed elsewhere. e.g., to heart and muscles, digestive system, menstrual flow, pregnancy.	Work at lower level. Avoid eating before exercise. Adjust to body's needs.	Make sure your class members are well educated before beginning the exercise programme.
Stitch.	Holding breath. Muscle spasm. Intestine full. Too brief a warm up.	Encourage controlled breathing. Discourage eating before exercise. Thorough warmup.	Walk down gently. Breathe deeply and stretch arms high. Bend forward and breathe out.
Blisters.	Badly fitted shoes. Bare feet rubbing on shoes.	Soak feet. Apply antiseptic cream. Cover the blister while exercising.	Make sure shoes fit properly. Wear socks.
Clicking joints	A variety of reasons which may be due to anatomical causes; can be serious or nothing to worry about.	If in pain check with a doctor or sports Injuries clinic.	Avoid hypertension of joints.
Stress incontinence.	Weak pelvic floor muscles. Prevalent in women after child birth or later in life.	Don't exercise with a full bladder. Avoid extreme jumping.	Good pelvic floor exercises will improve muscle tone and control
Muscle soreness and muscle strains.	Working too hard. Build up of lactic acid. Beginner to exercise. Muscular response to unfamiliar activity. Small muscle tears.	Adequate warm up. Always release after contraction to give a compensatory effect. Build up programme intensity slowly. Static stretches in cool down.	Massage. Alternate hot and cold bathing of affected part. Static stretches.
Knee pain.	Misalignment of body during exercise. Weak quadriceps muscles.	Wear good supporting footwear. Check alignment	Ensure good posture. Strengthen quadriceps. Work on alignment.
Back pain.	Overuse injury over a period of time.	Work at low level in aerobic section. Low level in abdominal work.	Strengthen back muscles. Smooth transition in level changes

The procedures for 'action in an emergency' are clearly set out in the authorised manual of St John Ambulance, which should be obtainable from your local St. John Ambulance representative, in case you need help, and to leave with him details of the location and times of your classes. It is also recommended that you know which of your local general practitioners is on call at the time of classes.

The most common incidents occurring in an exercise class include acute soft tissue injuries, where the muscle has torn causing sudden pain, inflammation and swelling, ankle sprains; or any sort of bruising resulting from a forceful impact. The following formula (RICE) will be the correct management for any of these.

R.I.C.E. – Rest, Ice, Compression, Elevation

Rest. The injured person should immediately discontinue the activity and be seated or lie down off the floor.

Ice. Apply a cold pack in the form of cold water, ice pack wrapped in a towel or gel cold pack. This has the effect of constricting the blood supply, decreasing the inflammation and numbing pain. Do not apply ice directly to skin as it can burn.

Compression. Wrap a bandage evenly and not too tightly around the ice pack, as this will help to limit the swelling.

Elevation. Place the injured limb at a higher level than the heart, to prevent blood 'pooling'.

Fractures, Dislocations, Bleeding

The RICE procedure should not be used for suspected fractures, dislocations or bleeding.

Where bones or joints may appear to be damaged or there is bleeding, the injured party will be in a state of *shock,* the signs of which will include: pallor, shallow breathing, rapid pulse, cold clammy skin.

First Aid Procedure.
1. The injured person should be laid down with legs elevated if possible.
2. Keep the person warm and as comfortable as possible.
3. Reassure him/her at frequent intervals in a calm manner
4. Control any bleeding with a sterile cloth applied with pressure.
5. If there is apparent deformity of the limb or joint avoid moving it as much as possible.
6. Call the ambulance immediately.
7. Make sure the person is accompanied to hospital.

Fainting

In cases of apparent fainting, the aim is to help the person regain consciousness by returning the flow of blood to the brain. Leaning forward with head on the knees will assist this process. Loosening tight clothing, reassurance and sips of cool water will all help to restore normality.

Severe Emergencies

Severe emergencies such as collapse may indicate heart attack or stroke and need immediate treatment in hospital. It may, however, be a good idea for the instructor to familiarise him/herself with the 'Save a Life' techniques, for which there are courses of instruction available in most localities.

Exercise note:
Recovery and return to exercise.
During the recovery period, the injured limb may need attention from a trained

physiotherapist who will recommend gentle stretching exercises to aid recovery. There is no reason to stop exercising other parts of the body if this does not affect the convalescent part. Return gradually to the full programme of exercise, building up strength in the muscles which support the damaged part. Test the injured part carefully before you fully extend its movement activity.

Long Term Overuse Injury

This type of exercise injury occurs slowly over time and is the result of an overload in endurance-type exercise, brought on by repetitive low-level stress to a body part. An extreme example of such overload would be jogging on a very hard floor surface in bare feet and landing incorrectly over a continous period.

Instructor's safety check

Common injuries of this type, which can arise from aerobic dance exercise and, in particular, jogging, are *shin splints* or, more seriously, *stress fractures*..

Shin splints:
An umbrella term for several conditions of the lower leg which give a great deal of pain after exercise. For example:

1. Muscles are contained within 'compartments' surrounded by a septum, or sheath. When the muscle pumps and swells up from activity such as jogging, which increases the blood supply to the muscle, there is expansion within the compartment. Too much muscle squeezed within a small compartment may give rise to pain.

2. The bones are covered with a fine membrane, the periosteum, which is supplied with nerve endings. A condition known as periosteal lifting can occur where repeated muscular contraction tugs at the attachments of muscle to bone and literally lifts the periosteum away from the bone.

Stress fractures:
These can occur when the bone is subjected to too much concussion. They can take the form of a hairline fracture of the tibia or fibula, torn ligament pulling off the bone and taking fragments of bone with it, or a full fracture of the bone.

Reasons for occurrence:
1. Incorrect floor surfaces.
2. Incorrect footwear.
3. Bouncing on the spot for long periods.
4. Weak arch of the foot.
5. Poor body control and alignment
6. Insufficiency of blood supply resulting from inadequate warm up exercises.

Prevention:
1. Improve the muscular balance in the lower leg: stretch the calf and strengthen the shin muscles.
2. Build up the tolerance of the tibia and fibula to concussive work in a progressive programme.

Treatment
1. Complete rest
2. Massage with ice – for shin splints only, *not* fractures.
3. Change to a non-weight-bearing aerobic activity.

Summary of Safety Measures

1. Pre-screening class members.
   Keep records, update and check out newcomers.

2. Monitor pulse rate.
   Interpret and evaluate information, and educate class members.

3. Favourable environment.
   Clothing, footwear, temperature, floor surface.

4. Design of programme
   Benefits and risks.

5. Controversial exercises.
   Avoid overload type of exercise causing stress and resulting in overuse injury.

6. First aid procedures.
   Basic emergency treatment; local medical resources.

Finally, there are two formal procedures it is advisable for every class instructor to follow:

1. Keep an Accident Record Book, logging dates and times of any accidents, names of injured parties and procedures taken.
2. Insure yourself for personal accident and, if working in a freelance capacity, make sure that you have a Public Liability insurance to give you legal cover in case of accident to a member of the public in your class who may sue for damages.

SECTION FIVE

Class Design

Aerobic dance exercise is for health-conscious people who want to get fit and stay fit. The promotion of this state of health-related fitness, rests with the instructor's ability as a communicator, to create a learning situation which is both motivating and rewarding to the participants.

This section is concerned with an understanding of the *Health* and *skill*-related components of physical fitness, and their incorporation in the design and structure of the exercise programme. It examines effective teaching methods and personal presentation skills, together with the administrative details of running a class.

Components of Fitness

Just as there is no single – universally accepted definition of physical fitness, there is also no universally accepted agreed list of physical fitness components. However, certain elements can be defined as representative of physical fitness, some of which are easy to measure and can be categorised. Definitions of the following components of physical fitness are adapted from 'Developmental Objectives of Physical Education' by A. Annarino; *Journal of Health, Physical Education and Recreation*, 1970, Vol. 41.

Organic Fitness

The first element of fitness is classified as *organic,* and is concerned with the proper functioning of the body systems so that the individual may adequately meet the demands placed upon him by his environment. This classification identifies the organic or health related components of physical fitness as follows:

Muscle strength. The maximum amount of force exerted by a muscle or muscle groups. The force effectiveness of localised muscle groups can vary, for example arm muscles can be weak and leg muscles strong.

Exercise note:
Muscle strength can be improved by resistance training, i.e., working against gravity, using own body weight as resistance or adding an external weight to load the body.

NB The aim should be to develop an optimum level of strength which enables the individual to cope with the demands of environment and working life without feeling overtired.

Muscle endurance, i.e., the ability of the muscle or muscle groups to sustain effort for a prolonged period of time. This involves a muscle performing a movement many times, building its stamina, without fatigue.

Muscular endurance is improved by increasing the number of repetitions of an exercise. There is need for release at regular intervals to avoid the build up of lactic acid if the muscle is working anaerobically.

NB The aim should be a gradual increase of tolerance to exercise repetition, building up muscular endurance to give general improvement in muscle tone over a period.

Cardiovascular endurance, i.e., the capacity of an individual to persist in strenuous activity for periods of some duration. This is dependent upon the combined efficiency of the blood vessels, heart and lungs.

Exercise note:
Aerobic exercise activity, which is continuous exercise for periods of 20-30 minutes and involves the use of large muscle groups, causes stress to the heart, lungs and circulatory system, accelerating their functions and raising the body's metabolic rate.

NB The aim should be to improve the overall efficiency of the cardiovascular system, at rest and during exercise, through a regular programme of aerobic exercise taken at spaced intervals, at least three times per week.

Flexibility, i.e., the range of movement in joints required to produce efficient body movement and minimise injury. Some joints are less flexible than others as a result of their anatomical structure, and are restricted by the supporting ligaments and tendons.

Exercise note:
The flexibility of the joints can be improved through stretching. Holding a static stretch for up to 30 seconds extends the range of movement in the joint over a period of time.

NB The aim should be to improve the general mobility of the body, keeping muscles supple and improving the range of movement.

Neuromuscular Fitness

The second element of fitness to be classified is *neuromuscular* and is concerned with the harmonious functioning of the nervous and muscular systems to produce desired movements. This classification identifies the neuromuscular or skill related components of physical fitness. The motor factors required for skill-related activities are:

Agility, i.e., the ability to change the level and direction of body movement with control.

Balance, i.e., the ability to maintain a static and dynamic equilibrium of the body parts and of the body as a whole.

Power, i.e., the ability to effect the optimal level of force in muscle groups over a minimum time period.

Reaction time, i.e., the ability to select a neuromuscular response with a minimal time delay, changing the response at intervals.

Speed, i.e., the ability to perform selected movements quickly and sustain the rate of performance.

Coordination, i.e., the ability to perform a range of movements with kinesthetic awareness, combining movements with accuracy, rhythm and timing, in a continuous sequence.

Some of the skill-related activities which contain these motor factors are both *locomotor*, e.g., walking, skipping, leaping, jumping, sliding, pushing, stepping, running, jogging, galloping, hopping, rolling, pulling, and *non-locomotor*, e.g., swaying, twisting, shaking, stretching, swinging, bending, lifting, stooping, curling. Both these skill-related activities are suitable for inclusion in the dance exercise programme.

Interpretive, Social and Emotional Fitness

Three further elements of fitness related to physical education contain objectives worthy of inclusion in the dance exercise programme:

Interpretive fitness, i.e., a knowledge of how the body functions and its relationship to physical activity.

Exercise note:
This kind of information can be acquired as a by-product of participation in class activity. A good instructor can feed interesting facts and information to class members, either overtly through visual data (posters/magazine articles), or more subtly by introducing topics of general interest for discussion at the end of class activities.

Social fitness, i.e., an adjustment to both self and others by an integration of the individual with society and his/her environment.

Exercise note:
The instructor can try to create a good class atmosphere within which each member will develop a sense of belonging to the group and identify with the common goal of achieving fitness.

Emotional fitness, i.e.,
1. A healthy response to physical activity through a fulfilment of basic needs.
2. The release of tension through suitable physical activities.
3. The ability to have fun!

Objectives of the Programme

The objectives of the dance exercise programme need, therefore, to be concerned with both physical response and mental attitude – a harmony of mind and body. Instructors should be aware of having an overall aim – the focal point towards which the effectiveness of the class as an experience of physical and mental fitness, is directed. The aim should be to develop within each individual a respect for their own bodily person, and in so doing, encourage a feeling of responsibility for personal maintenance. This will be fostered by a knowledge and understanding of the body, an appreciation of the significance of movement and last, but probably most important, an enjoyment of physical activity.

Structure of the Exercise Programme

For the class to be both safe and effective, all the components of physical fitness need to be contained within a well-structured programme. The programme should be designed to have a logical progression of movement and to be developmental, allowing for movement activity at beginner, intermediate and advanced levels.

A generally accepted format for the design of class activities is outlined below.

Programme Structure   *Duration:*   1 hour

1. Pre-class instruction   *3 minutes*
Take resting heart rate (RHR) pulse.

2. Warm-up   *8-10 minutes*
A balanced combination of rhythmic limbering exercises and static stretching, which alerts mind and body to activity.

Followed by specific areas of functional attention.

Head and neck
Shoulder girdle
Arms and chest/waist work
All best performed standing
for continuity
Hips/pelvic area
Legs/ankles/feet

Take training heart rate (THR) pulse, which should be raised within target zone.

3. Aerobic section   *20 minutes*
Take THR pulse, which should be maintained within target zone.

4. Warm down   *7 minutes*
Fairly lengthy, walking down, rhythmical movement to slow down the body.
Take RHR pulse, which should be within 20 beats of normal.

5. Body conditioning   *10-15 minutes*
Training muscular strength and endurance.
Often done as floor work.

6. Cool down   *5 minutes*
Slow static stretches.
Check RHR if desired.

This format may not always be possible if it is incompatible with the practicalities of class management. There may be external factors which dictate otherwise, such as time/ recreational breaks/caretaker, etc. However, certain 'Golden Rules' must be observed.

Four Golden Rules:

1. Always begin with a warm-up.
2. Always follow the aerobic section with sufficient warm-down.
3. Always, after conditioning muscles, stretch briefly to compensate before continuing to next group.
4. Always end the class with static stretching.

The percentage of time allocated to each section of the programme (based on a class at intermediate level) should be:

Warm up – 12 per cent
Aerobic – 40 per cent
Warm down – 10 per cent
Body conditioning – 30 per cent
Cool down – 8 per cent

1. *Body conditioning centred*
   Warm up 15 minutes
   Body conditioning 30 minutes
   Warm down/stretch 15 minutes

2. *Dance exercise centred*
   Warm up 20 minutes
   Dance steps and sequence 20 minutes
   Warm down/stretch 20 minutes

Two other invariables, essential to good class procedures, are pre-class screening and monitoring the heart rate.

Sequencing of Programme Activity

The actual sequence of exercise has its own logical progression to give adequate preparation and a good balanced arrangement of movement activity that is physiologically correct. The usual recommended sequence of activity is as follows.

Warm-up/Phase 1
Purpose: To prepare the body for the more strenuous work to follow. It should raise the heart rate, gradually increasing the cardiac output, and lubricate the joints, gently increasing mobility. It should also 'wake-up' the person mentally to a concentration on movement activity.

Fitness components: Flexibility/ cardiovascular output.

Activities. Locomotor: swinging/swaying/ lifting/walking/shaking. Non-locomotor: static stretches.

Body part involved: whole body; all major muscle groups.

Exercise Note:
This first part of warming up should not be too complex in design. Simple repetition and concentration on rhythmical, easy use of the body will be more beneficial than complicated sequences.

Warm-up/Phase 2
Purpose:– To extend the range of movement throughout the body and to raise the heart rate further to within the target zone. There should be a logical progression through the parts of the body from head to toe.

Fitness components:– Cardiovascular endurance/muscular endurance.

Activities:– Locomotor and non-locomotor.

Body parts involved:–
1. Head and neck (suboccipital group)
2. Shoulder girdle, chest and arms (trapezius, deltoid, biceps, triceps, pectoralis major.)
3. Rib cage, waist, lower back (external oblique, latissimus dorsi)
4. Groin area (hip flexors)
5. Thigh area (quadriceps, hamstrings, hip adductors, gracilis)
6. Calf muscles, front leg (gastrocnemius, soleus, tibialis anterior)
7. Feet and ankles (tibialis anterior, tibialis posterior, peroneus, long flexors and extensors of the toes)

It is possible to reverse the sequence and work from feet to head, but to maintain a smooth, coordinated flow from one area to another, avoid dodging about. It is also probably better to keep this part of the programme as 'standing' exercises, to maintain the preparatory feel of the body for the next phase. Particular attention should be given to warming the mobilising legs, feet and ankles thoroughly before aerobic activity.

Aerobic Phase

Purpose:– To strengthen the heart, improve the efficiency of the circulatory system and lungs, to exercise the large muscle groups and activate the metabolism to burn up calories.

Fitness components:– Cardiovascular endurance/skill-related (neuro-muscular) components.

Activities:– Non-locomotor (upper body and arm movements); locomotor (jogging, skipping, hopping, jumping, stepping, kicking, travelling).

Body parts involved:– Mainly concentrated on feet, ankles and calves with additional movements in shoulder girdle and arms.

The sequence of activities in this part of the programme should be built up slowly, so that participants feel confident, enjoy the movements and pick them up easily rather than experience frustration. This also gives time to adjust bodily and to cope with the increased demands placed on the physiological systems. Most people, other than trained dancers, have difficulty in coping with the motor factors of agility, balance, speed, reaction time and coordination: these are the skill-related components of fitness which have to be acquired through practice. So, build up the sequences of movement little by little, until final combinations of feet, arms, changes of direction and timing are achieved.

Remember that the aerobic phase needs to be geared to cope with three levels of participation – beginner, intermediate or advanced because of varying levels of fitness within the class. The instructor must plan the content of the programme at three levels and be prepared to demonstrate all three levels to encourage individual choice.

Duration. The length of the aerobic phase can be 20-30 minutes, but beginners can be encouraged to 'walk down' to a low level and just 'tick over' for some of the time. Maintaining the activity at a lower intensity will build up aerobic capacity; stopping suddenly is injurious.

Intensity can also be lowered by lessening the extent of other arm and body movement. This places less strain on the heart and keeps the heart rate within the target zone. Conversely, a more advanced student who has not managed to raise the heart rate sufficiently can increase the intensity by extending the range of movement to work harder. For example:

Low level: springy walking on spot/small steps/small or no arm movement/less power.

Intermediate: low level jog, toes just off floor/

bigger steps/moderate arm movements/increased power.

Advanced: high level jog, heels raised high/high lifting, deeper and wider steps/vigorous arm movements/maximum power.

Warm down

Purpose: Essential as a recovery from the strenuous aerobic phase, restoring normality, bringing the heart rate down slowly and helping to prevent the venous pooling of blood in the lower limbs.

Activities: The movements should be similar to the Warm up, but performed at a slower pace. They should feel relaxed and finally involve stretching in the lower limbs.

Body Conditioning

Purpose: These exercises are designed to overload the large muscle groups, training muscular strength and endurance. They should include both localised muscles and larger muscle groups.

Fitness components: Muscular strength/muscular endurance.

Activities: Non-locomotor.

Body parts involved: Hips/pelvic area (hip flexors, hip extensors, abductors, adductors) Buttocks (gluteus maximus, minimus and medius) upper and lower leg (quadriceps, hamstrings/gastrocnemius, soleus, tibialis anterior) Abdominals (rectus abdominis, external and internal obliques) Waist/arms, if not already covered (biceps, triceps/transverse muscles)

Exercise note:

Devising suitable exercises for this part of the programme requires an accurate knowledge of the muscle groups involved and an understanding of how to train strength and endurance. As a general rule:

★ If the exercise is difficult to do, e.g., press ups, it will probably only be sustained for a minimal number of repetitions and will therefore develop strength.

★ If the exercise is less difficult to do, e.g., abduction of the leg, it will probably be sustained for many more repetitions and will therefore emphasize endurance.

Abdominals

The muscles of the spine, buttocks and abdominal area work very much together, and a weakness in one will affect the others. Weak abdominals may mean back pain, as may weak buttocks and back muscles. When abdominal exercises are too strong, a dangerous strain will be placed on the back. Instead of the effort being placed on the rectus abdominis, it will also be taken by the hip flexors; the pelvis will rotate forward and the lower back will arch.

Abdominal muscles do not work as single muscles, but rather by the main direction of muscle fibres within the group. To train a sheet of muscle effectively, making it stronger and tighter, four exercises are needed which match the main directions of the fibres. These are:

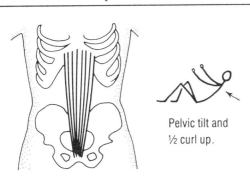

Pelvic tilt and ½ curl up.

1. Rectus Abdominis – Straight up and down in front

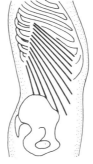

Side stretches

2. External obliques – Straight up and down at each side.

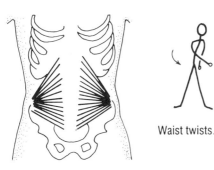

Waist twists.

3. Internal obliques – In opposite directions in front and around sides.

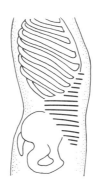

Diagonal waist twists or curl up.

4. Transversus Abdominis – Compression – narrowing in all directions

Lower limb
Awareness of the complexity of the knee joint is important, bearing in mind the stresses and strains put on this joint by weight bearing and locomotion. Exercises involving the knee must strengthen the quadriceps and hamstrings to help provide a strong, functioning stable joint. Thigh muscles need to be strong to maintain good posture in standing and walking. The muscles of the lower leg and foot are very important in support, propulsion and standing.

Buttocks
Exercises for the buttocks generally focus on the gluteal muscles and hamstrings and are usually executed in two ways:

1. Lying on the floor, knees bent – tilt pelvis and raise slightly off the floor, squeeze and lift, release and lower.

2. On hands and knees – lower and lift an extended leg keeping the horizontal line of the body and squeezing the buttock.

In both exercises, care should be taken not to overarch the lower back.

Finally: in all exercise where effort to promote strength or sustain a movement is required, remember to breath *out* for the difficult part of the exercise, and *in* for the recovery.

(Remember that it will be inappropriate to exercise the same muscle groups again, and allow for a release.

Cool Down

The final part of the programme emphasizes flexibility and mobility of joints and suppling of muscles. Static stretching should be smooth, slow and sustained. Stretches can be held for up to 30 seconds and should never be painful. It is important to stretch the muscle groups that have previously been contracted strongly, to give a compensatory effect. This conclusory phase should emphasize slow, controlled breathing to give a sense of refreshment and complete relaxation.

Instructional and Presentational Skills

The essential requirement for a clearly defined programme is a set of guidelines that act as a point of reference. Because of the many factors involved in selecting appropriate movement activity, it is more than useful to keep a written record of class activity each week. This should be aimed at showing different levels of progression – a graded programme to suit individual levels of fitness.

The Record Sheet

A record sheet should not only set out the exercise activity, but also analyse which muscle groups are involved and what fitness component is to be trained. This initial perspective provides the exercise with three dimensions, giving a picture of the relationship between *anatomy* (what body part?) *skill* (which locomotor or non-locomotor activity?) and *fitness component* (purpose of the exercise). This kind of analysis is useful in showing the overall balance of the programme. For example, it may be heavily weighted towards movement activity which strengthens and trains muscular endurance, with very little flexibility.

It is also a good idea to record any coaching points or areas of special concern and to note down the music used. Keeping a file of record sheets will provide a log book of class design for continual reference.

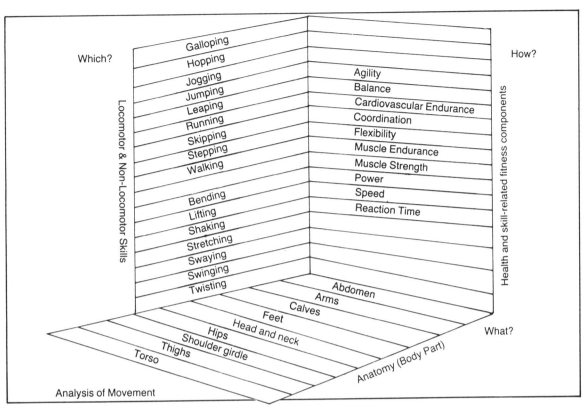

Which?

How?

Locomotor & Non-Locomotor Skills

Health and skill-related fitness components

Galloping
Hopping
Jogging
Jumping
Leaping
Running
Skipping
Stepping
Walking

Bending
Lifting
Shaking
Stretching
Swaying
Swinging
Twisting

Agility
Balance
Cardiovascular Endurance
Coordination
Flexibility
Muscle Endurance
Muscle Strength
Power
Speed
Reaction Time

Abdomen
Arms
Calves
Feet
Head and neck
Hips
Shoulder girdle
Thighs
Torso

Analysis of Movement

What?

Anatomy (Body Part)

Record Sheet:	Class:					No.			
	Activity	Muscle group	Fitness component	Coaching point	Beginner	Level Inter-mediate	Advanced	Music
Pre-class Instruction								
Warm Up								
Aerobic Section								
Warm Down								
Body Conditioning								
Stretch Cool Down								
Comments								
Evaluation								

Bearing in mind the need for graded progression, it is possible to aim the class at an intermediate level, with an option up to advanced or down to beginner level.

Beginners:

1. Keep activity at a low level:
   A long warm up
   Shorter aerobic section (monitor pulse rates at least twice)
   Lower intensity body conditioning
   Long stretch and cool down

2. Thoroughly coach foot work in jogging activity:
   Weight taken through toe, ball, heel in on-the-spot dance activity
   Running forward changes to heel, ball, toe

3. Constant observation of danger zones:
   Neck, spine, hips, knees, ankles

4. Correct posture and alignment:
   Coach body carriage and control in jogging

5. When planning movement activity, AVOID:
   Balancing on one foot, until the ankles are strong
   Diagonal work, until alignment is sound
   Multidimensional travelling, as it can be confusing and lead to loss of body control
   Heavy back and knee work, danger zones
   High or heavy arm work which is stressful to cardiovascular system
   Deep plies, which cause stress to joints unless thighs are strong and posture good
   Too many repetitions: this must be built up slowly
   Holding positions for too long. Overstretching can cause damage until greater flexibility is gained.

Exercise note:

Assuming that the class is working at an intermediate level (and many of the class members will be quite happy to maintain this pace) it is important not to forget that there will probably be a nucleus of people who have attended class for some time and will have a higher level of fitness. They will quickly become bored if they are not given a progression which challenges their physical working capacity.

For advanced work:
   Increase the number of repetitions.
   Increase the range of motion.
   Add stronger arm movements to leg work.
   Provide a longer aerobic section.
   Change the leverage to make the body work harder.
   Increase the complexity of the exercise.
   Work with added wrist or ankle weight.

This progressive overload should be introduced gradually – not everything at once – to bring about a greater achievement over time.

Evaluation

If teaching the exercise programme is to be an on-going process, there will be need for adjustment, change and development, both in programme content and possibly in the teaching approach. The record sheet provides a space for comment and an assessment of progress, successes and failures, which can provide a basis for future development. Such an evaluation of the programme helps the instructor to learn from the mistakes or build on the successes and so generally improve on what has gone before.

An aid to this evaluative process is one of the most important instructional skills a teacher can possess – the power of *observation*. Fundamental to this role of observer is the ability to watch with a keen awareness, i.e., to scan the whole class but also be alert to each member, and in so doing to make an accurate appraisal of the movement techniques demonstrated by every member of the class. Given the guidelines that the instructor has set for the movement activity, he/she will be looking for cues or pointers indicating that certain criteria are not being met and variations of the movement are being performed.

Have a thorough and accurate understanding of the specification of the exercise activity, i.e.:

    Fitness component
    Body part
    Skill activity
    Purpose (where the activity occurs in the programme)
    Possible dangers – Vulnerable body areas
                                Posture and alignment
                                Approach to recovery from the
                                exercise
    Level – Beginner/Intermediate/Advanced

It should be possible for the instructor to anticipate the possible errors and use the pre-class instruction time to coach procedures for the correct execution of an exercise. Taking a different coaching point each week will gradually build up the class knowledge of correct technique.

Observational techniques
1. Scan the class rapidly while instructing to try to identify people's names mentally. Note their capability for future reference.

2. Anticipate potential error and coach accordingly.

3. Change position of observation – side or rear view – or move among the class.

4. Know the newcomers and beginners and check their progress.

5. Never teach totally with your back toward the class. Look through to the back of the class for members who may be out of view and become an unknown quantity. People tend to keep a favourite spot: some may never be seen and so are always overlooked.

6. Always make sure that the class is positioned in the best possible way for safe execution of the exercise, and to see and be seen.

7. Learn to be the mirror for the class, indicating right and left side correctly.

Methods of correction

1. Point out errors in a general way and coach as you go along.

2. Never single out individual mistakes.

3. Individual correction should be discreet – stand at side and show correct movement. Avoid passive (physical adjustment) which may be harmful or even offensive. A light touch or adjustment to body position is acceptable.

Personal Presentation

Alongside the teacher's skill in instructional techniques, and closely allied to it, is the method of presentation. Presentation of the 'perfect image' has been the somewhat narcissistic impression reflected by the 'gurus' of the fitness industry. Personal standards of excellence in technique and accurate demonstration of exercise activity are important, even essential, to raise the standards of class members, who must have a model to copy and are aspiring to better their own performance. However, perhaps because of the advent of the mirrored studio, many teachers fall into the trap of becoming so wrapped up in their own performance that they fail to give adequate time and space to translating their skills into a practical and informative movement vocabulary that class members can understand. A good instructor must relate personal competence through clear methods of instruction and presentation, to provide an agreeable climate of learning within which class members feel a sense of achievement and motivation, rather than frustration and withdrawal.

Good presentation of the exercise programme to the class requires of the instructor an appearance, attitude and demeanour that convey a commitment to a healthy lifestyle and an enthusiasm for fitness. He/she should also appear confident and give the impression of being in command.

To provide sound instruction the instructor needs the ability to structure the order and sequence of programme material according to the needs and interests of the class and to convey the aims of the programme through his/her teaching.

Structure of Teaching

This will probably be dictated by the teaching situation. A large class lends itself to a more formal structure, particularly if there is a restriction on time.

Formal, teacher-directed (passive) learning. In this situation the instructor directs and controls the group, and sets the movement tasks to be accomplished in a given time. The class listens, assimilates and responds. The instructor sets the pace and keeps the class fairly rigidly within the guidelines, tending not to deviate, although alterations can be made to allow for the slowest members.

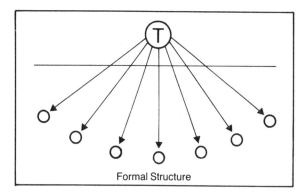

Formal Structure

Teacher directed (autocratic) Passive learning. This style of teaching will be more comfortable for the inexperienced instructor, who has not yet evolved a personal style.

Informal, teacher and task-centred (active) learning. A more informal teaching structure may be possible where the group is smaller, for example, up to 20 people. In this situation the instructor is a member of the group, but still the expert. He/she helps the group towards achieving the movement tasks, with class members taking a more active part in class design. This type of teaching provides more awareness of individual needs through the opportunity to change the class structure, and greater interaction between instructor and class.

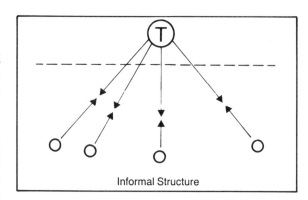

Informal Structure

Verbal Communication Skills

Presentation

1. Qualities in voice production are clarity and good articulation, with adequate projection. Check the acoustics and make sure you can be heard over the music.

2. Lower the pitch and tone of the voice and make it interesting by altering the intonation. This can help to emphasize a required aspect of the movement activity, and also to motivate greater effort.

Instruction

1. Be concise to be effective. Give the correct information: don't say one thing and do another.

2. Coach and instruct the class through the progression of the exercise, counting beats, and giving cue words, e.g., 1, 2, stretch high; 5, 6, and repeat.

3. Mention the salient points which need careful execution.

4. Count through the number of repetitions and give cues for the changeover from right to left, before the actual change, so that people are not left behind.

Non-Verbal Communication Skills

A certain amount of non-verbal communication can establish a good relationship and interaction between class and instructor:

Establish eye to eye contact
Look at individual class members
React to class needs and be sensitive to class response
Observe people's body language, indifference, boredom, fatigue, enjoyment, enthusiasm
Smile and show how you feel with facial expressions of sympathy, amusement, surprise.

Demonstration Technique

Presentation

1. Good posture, alignment, body control and movement technique should be representative of the highest standards of excellence the instructor can achieve.

2. Practice the execution of movements beforehand, preferably in front of a mirror.

3. Know exactly what is required in terms of body mechanics, relationship of body parts and distribution of weight.

4. Be practised and precise with skill-related components of fitness (balance, agility, timing, coordination, rhythm and fluidity).

Instruction

1. Practical demonstration can be informal – follow the leader – the class picking up the sequence as they go along. This method suits the aerobic dance exercise class where continuity is required.

2. More specific illustration can be made to bring out coaching points, e.g.,
   Demonstrate the whole exercise
   Break it down and teach separate parts
   Put it back together, integrating parts
   Repeat with class, class repeats/instructor observes, or
   Use an assistant to demonstrate
   Instructor observes levels of ability while class repeats with assistant
   Instructor moves round class monitoring and correcting.

Class Management

If the first aim of the instructor is to encourage and foster health-related fitness as a way of life, the second and perhaps more selfish aim might be to ensure that his/her classes continue to grow in numbers and flourish in reputation.

The sense of motivation and purpose developed by participation in a class is a two way process: enthusiastic and motivated class members give back their enthusiasm and motivation to the instructor

All too often an initial enthusiasm for taking up an exercise activity will wane and the 'drop out' syndrome occurs. To avoid losing members of the class, the instructor must be constantly aware of the art of class management.

Good class management relies on the instructor's ability to direct and control events. The instructor is rather like the conductor of an orchestra, who brings together a great many skills to produce a worthwhile and satisfactory performance from each member of the group, at the same time creating total harmony.

Motivation

If the class is to have good pace and continuity, it is important that the instructor achieves a fine balance between the 'talking, demonstrating' and the class 'doing'. Too much passive watching, and the class will become bored, reluctant, uninterested and physically cold. Adults who have come back to a learning situation usually want to learn; bearing in mind that this is a recreative learning situation, they will still want to learn by 'doing' and taking an active part. A class member's motivation to continue to attend may largely be affected by how enjoyable the situation is for him/her, and this will be influenced by a sense of achievement obtained through active participation.

Fitness Goals

Another influencing factor in continuation of class attendance is whether, in the end, it is a worthwhile experience. Achieving the goals of health and skill-related fitness may depend on how skilful the instructor is at relating to her class and discovering their individual needs and hopeful outcome from the class. Informal discussion may reveal a class preference for more body conditioning or a longer aerobic section. In this case the instructor should not be afraid to adjust to the needs of the class, drop some activities and adopt others. Keeping a record of training heart rate levels and encouraging class members to develop a programme of fitness activity (e.g., aerobic dance exercise three times a week, at spaced intervals, to gain a minimum training effect) encourages a feeling of working toward an improved physical state.

Social Integration

A feeling of class unity can be encouraged by the sharing of fitness experiences. This can be introduced through informal discussion and helps the instructor to evaluate what the class likes or dislikes in exercise and how this fits in with the current programme of instruction. Taking part in demonstrations and displays in the local community also lends a corporate image to a group.

Evaluation

Looking at mistakes, reviewing and correcting will help the instructor to present a better programme, best suited to the needs of the class. Sensitivity to class preferences comes through observation and the establishment of channels of communication. Such channels provide a 'feedback' from the class which gives the instructor a better understanding of whether aims and objectives are being fulfilled.

Choreography and Dance

Dance trains the body to move expressively. It is this creative element which gives the Dance Exercise Programme its particular inventive form and style.

This section is concerned with the vocabulary of movement and technical skills that dance provides, the arrangement of movements to give patterns for action, and the use of music, its rhythms and phrasing, as an accompaniment to dance exercise.

Dance Movement Vocabulary

In its simplest form, dance is the body in motion, the nature of which is governed by the expressive use of the body. Dance training seeks to expand individual control and mastery of body manipulation in movement activity, in terms of weight, space and time. The understanding and correct application of these principles involve consideration of correct body alignment, the relationship and positioning of body parts, the distribution of body weight, the area which the movement encompasses and the speed and control with which the movement is executed.

The dance exercise programme has borrowed extensively from the specialised world of dance, combining elements from ballet, tap, jazz, modern stage and folk dance, to create interesting movement patterns and combinations. As a result the instructor will need to convey the underlying principles of dance technique to make sure that class members manipulate their bodies as safely as possible.

Skill-related activities require a great deal of body awareness and control to be executed correctly. Therefore, although a highly skilled performance is not necessarily the primary aim of a fitness class, to be safe and effective a certain amount of technical skill must be acquired.

Posture and Alignment

The most important area to consider is that of body posture. Good posture means correct alignment of body parts and distribution of weight, at rest and during activity.

Individual differences in environment and the various uses to which our bodies are put in everyday life result in the evolution of many different ways of handling the body posturally, both at rest and during activity. These vary from person to person, have become habitual for that person and feel correct. Each person evolves a postural stance

– a distinctive gait which identifies him as an individual and is part of his physical character. As a result many variations and postural differences exist between individuals. Some postures will inevitably reveal skeletal and muscular imbalance, causing the body to be mechanically inefficient, and even affecting physiological function. An instructor's first job is to establish a form of correct posture as a basis for movement activity, and to reinforce this throughout the teaching programme.

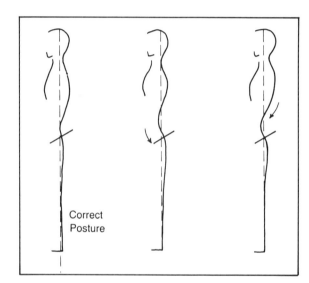

Correct Posture

The second sacral vertebra is approximately the centre of gravity of the body, and other body parts should be balanced in relation to this. Thus the line of gravity will fall in the centre of the very small base formed by the feet.

Deviation in one part of the body alters the alignment of the rest of the body in order to keep a balance and maintain the line of gravity within the base.

Posture in movement

Achieving a good static posture is a preparatory phase, leading to maintenance of good posture in movement. Movement is a series of connecting body positions which are linked posturally, each preceding posture facilitating the next one.

In good movement there is a harmonious relationship between the physiological function and the mechanics of the movement. The body position gives a sensory stimulus, via the nerves, from the joint capsule, ligaments and muscle, initiating an efficient muscular response and action. For the movement to be coordinated and executed

Instructor's safety check

	Bad Posture	Good Posture
Head Neck	Falls back or tucks forward Pokes up or down (hyperextended)	Feel hooked to ceiling through top of head Chin parallel to floor
Shoulders	Hunched forward or pressed back	Relaxed and square
Spine	Chest pushed out or caved in (rounded) (Lower back hyperextended)	Lengthened – upper back lifts and broadens Ribs lifted out of hips
Abdomen	Protrudes	Drawn in – flattened
Hips	Tilt or twist	Squared
Bottom	Pushed out	Pulled down, lengthened – gluteus maximus tightened
Thighs	Falling inward	Contracted muscles pulling up
Knees	Overtightened (locked joint), poorly aligned	Slightly relaxed, good alignment of knee and foot
Ankles	Rolling in or out	Held in centre
Feet	Weight in heels. Body off balance	Weight in balls of feet. Body balanced

with maximum efficiency, the body must be totally in tune. This requires training.

Exercise note:
Positioning of the feet is important at rest and in movement, and for the purpose of the dance exercise programme these are generally three foot placement positions, as shown:

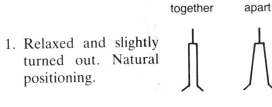

	Feet together	Feet apart

1. Relaxed and slightly turned out. Natural positioning.

2. Rotation out from the hip through knee and ankle joint. Ballet turn out through an angle of up to 180°.

3. Parallel position. Feet pointing straight forward.

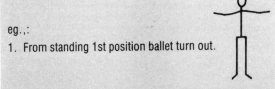
Body Actions and Dance Steps

The non-locomotor activities, which include all non-weight-bearing movements, are likely to be useful material for the warm up and warm down parts of the programme. Gestural movements that stretch, swing, lift, bend and twist the body will increase flexibility and mobility and can be rhythmically limbering in nature. The arms are the natural instigators of gestures into space and will lead the trunk and head into larger movements of the whole body.

A technique borrowed from jazz dance is isolation of body parts in movement. This technique trains the centres of movement – head, chest, shoulders, pelvis, arms and legs to achieve an independent mobility. Once the class has mastered the skills of isolation of body parts and can move them independently of each other, more sophisticated sequences can be structured by practising the movement using a combination of parts with coordinated working of two or more together. For example, practice independently:
1. Head turn right.
2. Right arm extended, palm forward; roll shoulder back and release, palm upward.
3. Move ribs to left.

Or in combination:
Turn head to right, at same time move ribs left and roll shoulder back, releasing palm upward.

Movement of the body through the surrounding space, with control and adjustment of speed, requires assimilation of a vocabulary of locomotor skill-related activities. Locomotor activities include stepping, travelling, jumping and turning, that is the skills which require balance, agility, coordination, speed, fast reaction and power. Most dance steps are built from these locomotor activities, and are a creative combination of step-movement patterns. This arrangement of movement activity, in particular, lends itself to the aerobic section of the dance exercise programme. Dance steps are an essential foundation for a provision of continuous sequence of movement, particularly if the focus is to be 'low impact', rather than 'high intensity'. A creative instructor will find an endless source of material here.

Identification of Movement Activities ★
Stepping Transference of weight, usually from one foot to another.
Travelling. Transference of weight in successive movement of body parts (e.g. feet/hands), one after the other to cover ground.
Jumping. Elevating the body away from the force of gravity.
Turning. Changing the body's front in movement.
Stillness. Holding a body position. This requires muscular tension and trains balance. It also emphasizes the relationship between the body parts.

★From *A Handbook for Modern Educational Dance*, V. Preston

Choreography for Dance Exercise

Choreography is a method of mapping out the movement to provide a pattern for action. The basic choreographic skills required for dance exercise are simple arrangements of steps and body activity into combinations and sequences. This involves division of movement activity, through timing, repetition, coordination of steps and movement of body parts, to build up a sequence.

The basis of dance technique is the ability of the body to move through sequences of activity skilfully. The following combined movement activities can be identified

1. Stepping with added gesture.
2. Stepping during locomotion.
3. Travelling and turning.
4. Turning jumps.
5. Gestures during jumps.
6. Gestures and locomotion.
7. Travelling jumps.
8. Step-jump rhythms.
9. Stepping during turns.
10. Turns with gestures.

Ideas for Dance Step Combination and Sequence:

Basic step	Variations
1. Step on to R foot. Close L foot and transfer weight.	Change direction, or number of repetitions. Change speed; add gesture with leg.
2. Step on to R foot. Touch L foot beside it. Step L foot-touch R foot.	Touch foot in front/behind/side. Step touch and step back with quarter or half turn and touch.
3. Step forward R foot. Keeping feet apart do half turn to face opposite direction. Transfer weight to L foot and repeat.	Pivot Weight on L foot – R leg extended, weight on ball of foot. Rotate the body to the right, transferring weight to R foot – bringing L foot in to touch. Rotation can be stopped at:

¼   ½   ¾   Full turn

4. Grapevine Cross R foot in front – step left. Cross R foot behind – step left. Cross R foot in front – step left. Cross R foot behind – swing L leg around to cross L foot and go back, reversing direction.	Hopping on one foot, flex heel and point toe of other foot. Repeat 4R/4L/2R/2L/1R/1L. Repeat turning in a square.
5. Ball change R Foot in front, weight forward – L foot behind, weight on ball of foot. Simple rapid weight transference – drop back on to L foot quickly and forward on R foot, Left and right.	Kick ball change: Swing and kick L foot first, and then ball change – transferring weight as before. Kick left and right. Add stepping:– step, step, kick, ball change. Direction:– Step, step, kick, ball change and turn to right. Complete a square, turning right. Repeat to left.
6. Jumping/hopping: There are five basic jumps: 1. One foot to same foot (hop) – levé. 2. One foot to other foot (leap) – jeté. 3. One foot to both feet – assemblé 4. From both feet to both feet – sauté. 5. From both feet to one foot – sissone.	Sequence Four small jumps forward. Four runs backward. Repeat sideways.
7. Step, step, step, hop change direction Run, run, run, hop turn in a square Spring from one foot to other – forward/back, side/side.	Hopping on one foot (not more than four times) while shaking other leg. Repeat round in square. Repeat 4R, 4L/2R, 2L/1R and 1L. Repeat turning in a square – heel and toe right, turning right. Heel and toe left, turning left.
8. Transfer weight from R to L foot in a sideways swinging movement.	Jump both feet to both feet – twist hips – or take feet apart and together.

Dance Stretches and Isolations

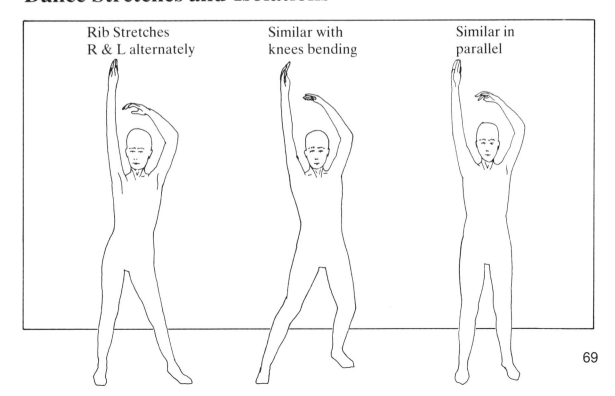

Rib Stretches
R & L alternately

Similar with
knees bending

Similar in
parallel

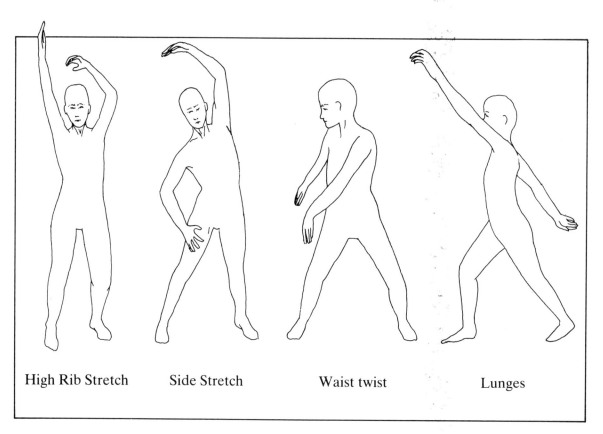

High Rib Stretch   Side Stretch   Waist twist   Lunges

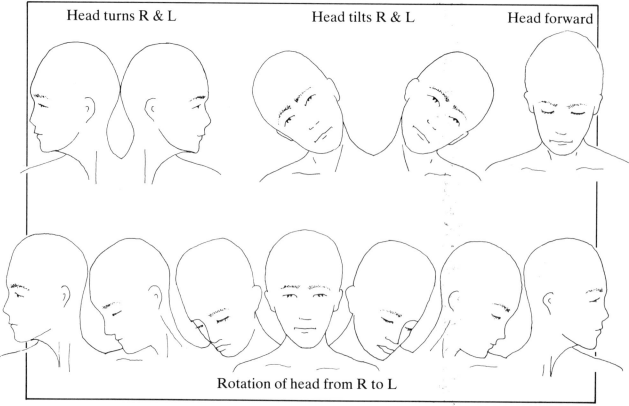

Head turns R & L   Head tilts R & L   Head forward

Rotation of head from R to L

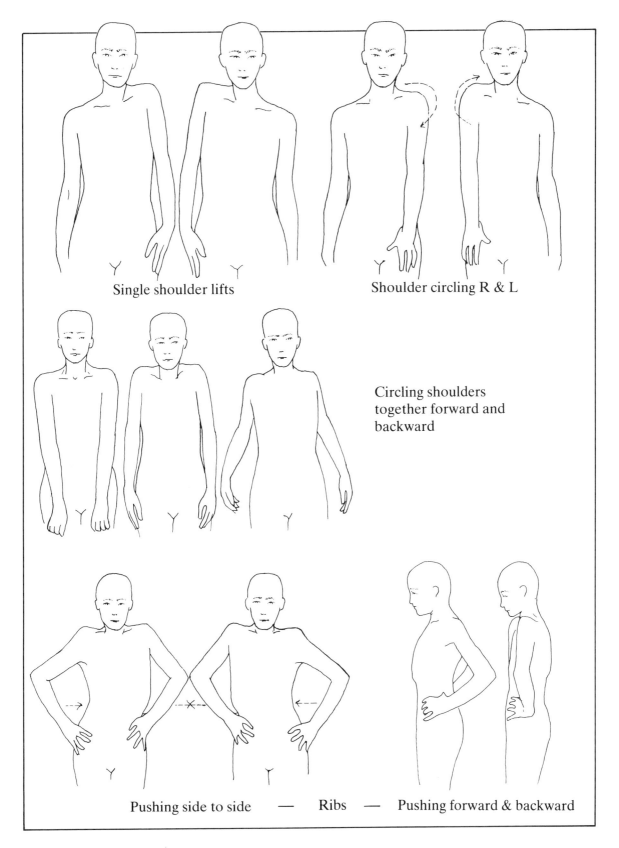

Single shoulder lifts

Shoulder circling R & L

Circling shoulders together forward and backward

Pushing side to side — Ribs — Pushing forward & backward

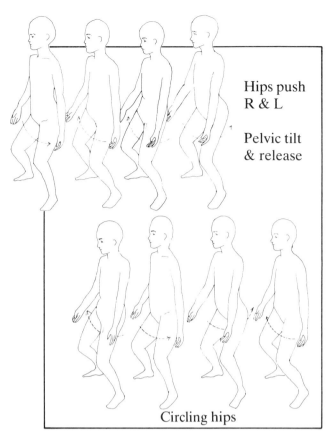

Hips push
R & L

Pelvic tilt
& release

Circling hips

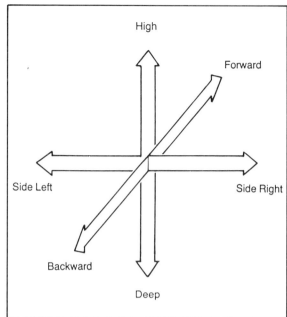

Combinations of dance steps into these six dimensions will provide many variations for patterns of movement.

Use of Space

Once the body moves off the spot, it moves into and through the surrounding space while still retaining its own personal sphere of space, which is bounded by the limits of the body's range of motion. The body can reach into space in different directions and can also travel into space in different directions. Dividing the surrounding spatial areas into sections gives form and structure to movement choreography.

Considering the level at which the body can move gives three dimensions, high, medium and deep, open to exploration. Moving fully into each dimension, or combining movements from one to the other will extend the body's range of motion. Movements can also be made up or down, from side to side, or forward and back. Therefore, movement can be achieved in six dimensions which diagrammatically form a cross.

Instructor's safety check:

Always build up multidimensional travelling sequences with added co-ordinated arm work very gradually. Start with the basic step and expand a little at a time. This is especially important for beginners.

e.g., Stepping sequence

1. Step right and left, transferring weight evenly, stretching leg forward and pointing toe.

2. Repeat with a slight spring from right to left, leaning back slightly.

3. Travel forward four and back four with this step.

4. Add both arms, lifting high on forward travel. Lower both arms behind hips on backward travel. (Maintain stretched leg, pointed toe.)

5. Repeat whole combination – forward/backward – turn right, until a square to the right is completed.

6. Repeat to the left in the same way.

★ From *A Handbook for Modern Educational Dance*, V. Preston Dunlop

Music

The dance exercise programme is essentially a programme of exercise set to music, and the musical component exerts a powerful influence. Music pervades our social and working hours as a background accompaniment and, as such, is an accepted part of everyday life. It is partly because of the combination of popular music with appropriate movement that the dance exercise programme set a new trend as a form of recreational fitness.

Music as an aid to exercise can be both motivating and emotive. It can make you want to move, and make you feel good while moving. It sets the pace and mood of an exercise sequence and adds variety to class activity. It provides cues for movement which help the instructor to know when to change the exercise or begin a new section, and these cues are passed on to the class. Music provides an enjoyable atmosphere, suggesting a happy class environment.

Components of Music

Music can be divided into the following four components:

Beat. The underlying defined and regular, predominant sound which gives the music its quality.

Metric rhythm. The reoccurrence of the beat at marked intervals, which accentuates the phrasing of the music and can be counted in groups, e.g., 2/4, 4/4, 3/4.

Speed. The rate at which the rhythm is played, e.g., half-time, single time or double time.

Tempo. The speed at which the music is played. This is determined by the metric quality, i.e., number of beats per minute, and can be slow-sustained, slow, medium or fast.

Selection and Organisation of Music

Bearing in mind that we live in an age of background music, music for the exercise class should be chosen with care. Consider first the age group, sex and occupations of class members, and how this may reflect their tastes in music. Also, if the instructor does not feel inspired by the music, it is unlikely that the class will!

Exercise note:
Who? An older group may respond to a more relaxed 'easy to move to' style, e.g., Country and Western, Ballads, Big Band style. A younger group will be more likely to enjoy current trends in popular music, e.g., Soul, Jazz, Rock, Reggae.

Setting the atmosphere through the choice of music creates a musical climate to suit the movement. What you do to the music may be governed by its speed, tempo and also the mood suggested by the lyrics or instrumental rhythms.

What? Warm up – medium tempo, 3/4 rhythm, energizing mood.
Warm down – medium tempo, 3/4 rhythm, relaxing mood.
Aerobic – fast tempo, 2/4 or 4/4 rhythm, good pace, motivating.
Body conditioning – slow temp, 4/4 rhythm, positive, definite beat.
Cool down – slow-sustained, 4/4 or 3/4 rhythm, soothing, relaxing.

Listening to and looking for suitable music as an accompaniment has to be a continuous process. Current popular music tends to change rapidly and it can be expensive to keep up to date. However, the instructor will need to change the music fairly regularly to cultivate a lively and varied class atmosphere.

Some music becomes 'classic', in that its popularity does not fade but becomes

1. 2/4 and 4/4 rhythms are easy to work with, as the movement can be divided into 2 or 4 parts, and 8-beat or 16-beat phrases are good lengths for repetition of an exercise.

2. If you are not confident about using several pieces of music put together in sequence, it is a good idea to begin with a continuous recording of the popular 'remix' type, as this obviates having to know where you are in the music. It provides a steady rhythmic and melodic background, and you can stop and start without losing the place.

3. Once you become more confident, put together several styles of music to give variety and interest to your class.

4. Different styles of music will emphasize the different sections of the programme and will help you to remember the sequence of movement.

5. Emphasize the strong movements that require increased effort by clapping or clicking fingers or beating hands to body, feet or floor, in time with the strong beat of the music.

6. Avoid music which changes speed or tempo suddenly or unexpectedly, or adds a beat, as this can throw the order of movement in the exercise sequence.

7. Too much vocal accompaniment may be distracting to the concentration required to follow the movement.

8. Make sure the music is not too loud and is positioned correctly so that you can be heard. Test this out with someone in class beforehand.

9. Don't be afraid to stop and start again if you begin badly and lose track of the sequence.

10. Always monitor the music level during the programme

    – Turn it down if you feel it is too loud.
    – Turn it up if it cannot be heard.
    – Turn it low or off to take the pulse.
    – Turn it off to coach or break down an exercise.

11. Playing background music before and after the programme makes class member feel 'at home' and is reassuring; people like to chat together and this is sometimes inhibited in a hushed silence.

established. This is true of modern as well as classical styles. Keeping a personal tape library of these classic favourites is a good practice, as they can be brought back into use from time to time and mixed with currently popular sounds. Libraries can be a source of music, and fellow instructors are usually willing to swap their music ideas.

However, it is a legal requirement that everyone who teaches an exercise class to music should hold a licence to do so. Fees vary with the type of class taught, number of people in the class and whether the class is termly or throughout the year. Evasion of purchase of this licence can lead to prosecution. (Licences in the UK can be obtained from Phonographic Performance Ltd., (PPL), Ganton House, 14-22 Ganton Street, London, W1 6LB. For other countries it is important to check licencing procedures).

Instructor's note:

1. Make sure you record on high quality chrome tape which is less likely to stretch or break.

2. Make two recordings so that you have a spare.

3. Tape each recording at the correct recording level to avoid distortion.

4. Write down the name of the record and recording artist on the cassette label and the section of the programme it is for.

5. Keep reference list of each cassette, number it and state which exercise programme it accompanies.

6. Work through your exercise programme without music, using vocal accompaniment.

7. Make a rough tape first, try out the sequence and make alterations.

8. Keeping pieces of music separately from the continuous programme tape is useful if the class has to be adapted suddenly. This saves running through the tape to look for music.

9. Always have your tapes set at the right place ready to start.

Combining Music with Movement

Working through set routines choreographed to fit set music is the framework of dance exercise. Having a good music 'sense' – an intuitive feel for the phrasing of the music is a valuable asset for the instructor and can be acquired with practice, if it is not a natural gift. Again, considerable time and practical application are required to become perfect.

Instructor's note:

1. Select music which appears suitable and listen through it several times.

2. Pick out the defined beat of the music.

3. Count out the beats in groups to establish the tempo. Once you have the count, clap it out.

4. Find the accented stronger beat in relation to the lighter beats.

5. Feel the rhythm of the music by moving the body. The music may suggest the type of movement. Keep it simple and repeat it in time on the spot.

6. Enlarge the movement by moving off the spot, still keeping time. Develop the sequence of movement with directional changes within the number of beats dictated by the music.

7. Talk through the movement, accentuating the cue words and coaching words, e.g.,
   And forward 2, 3, 4.
   And backward 2, 3, 4.
   Stretch 2, 3. *Change left* 2, 3.
   Step, step, step, *and hop.*

8. Practice these talking-through sessions with the music until you feel that they are fully integrated. The music should begin to 'suggest' the movement quality.

9. Make sure you have counted through the introduction. Use it for preparation for the exercise. Know when to start.

10. Use the voice over the music almost to sing along with the sound. Use voice intonation and pitch to pick out beat and rhythm and give emphasis to the movement.

11. Try to suit the dynamics of the music to the expression and mood of the movement, and try to match the musical motif with corresponding movement motifs, so that repetition of movement echoes through the music.

12. Listen to the accents – high spots, low points, syncopations, changes of tempo. Relate this to the type of movement.

Class Administration

Qualification

Before you set out to establish yourself as an instructor of dance exercise, it is important to obtain a valid qualification. There are many courses on the market which lead to qualification as a teacher of exercise, and they vary enormously both in cost and content. Before you part with any money, establish the criteria of the course: will it give a certification which is acceptable to local education authorities? Current plans for a scheme to give nationally recognised qualifications are underway. This involves the RSA (Royal Society of Arts) and the Sports Council drafting the outline of an assessment scheme, syllabus and moderation plan for a 'Certificate for Teachers of Exercise to Music'. Now this scheme has been launched, many existing courses will be able to apply for RSA validation if they meet the required standards, and there should no longer be any confusion over what is a recognised qualification.

Once qualified, a sense of professionalism requires that the instructor keep up to date in the subject, and this involves attending courses, lectures and workshops, reading up on current information and keeping in contact with other fitness teachers. Belonging to a professional association provides such opportunities and gives advice and support.

Setting up a Class

Location:

1. Discover a suitable location by walking round your selected area.

2. Find out which organisations already operate in that area. Is there competition?

3. Are there other existing groups, e.g., parents and toddlers, WI, Young Wives, over 60's? These are groups who may welcome a fitness class to add to their activities' list.

4. Look for sports centres, health clubs, squash, tennis or swimming clubs as possible sites for your class, because these are groups already committed to fitness.

5. If you decide to be independent, there are many halls which are available for hire at a reasonable rate.

6. Bear in mind that a daytime class may attract young mothers who need crèche facilities.

7. Check availability and times.

Equipment:

1. Make sure you own or have access to a reliable cassete recorder with good sound reproduction, which can be heard clearly in a large hall.

2. Make sure your tapes are well put together and that you have spares.

3. Plan the programme.

4. Design safety posters, screening chart and target zone chart.

5. Buy a small card filing system to index class members.

6. Collect resource material for class information.

7. Buy a stopwatch or have a wrist watch with clear second had.

Finance:

1. Having acquired the venue, check the legal aspects of setting up the class.

2. Find out if you are covered by the hiring authority or by club management for playing music to the public; if not, obtain a licence from PPL (see p.74)

3. Make sure that you have both personal insurance and public liability insurance to cover yourself in the event of accident or injury, to you or to a member of the public.

4. Make sure the project is financially viable by weighing up the initial outlay in expenditure, and the ongoing expenditure, with the amount you can reasonably expect to charge members.

5. Do you need to charge in advance for, say, a set of 6 classes or can you risk people paying week by week?

Advertisement:

1. Be enterprising with advertising procedures: local newspapers can be expensive.

2. Look for local advertising papers which can be cheaper.

3. Find out if the paper is doing a special feature on health and fitness.

4. Local church magazines will often include details of activities in the area.

5. Design an attractive poster, make photocopies, place in shops, library, clinics, local group meeting places.

6. Talk to people, interest them in the availability of the class and encourage them to tell their friends.

Class Procedures

1. Set out visual aid material, prepare equipment, check first aid equipment and emergency phone number(s).

2. Pre-screen each new member.

3. Introduce yourself, give information about the style of the class, how it operates, fitness goals and safety levels.

4. Try to gather information about the class as individuals and to assess their needs.

5. Monitor attendance and keep record files up to date; check drop out rate.

6. Set the learning climate of the class according to class needs and the fitness goals you have incorporated into the programme.

7. Monitor the class progress and individual members' progress, obtaining feedback through informal methods.

8. Evaluate your findings and, in the light of the information, be aware of adjustment and change that might need to be made.

Programme Plan for Aerobic Dance Exercise

Take Pulse to monitor Resting Heart Rate   **WARM UP:**

Sec	Fig no.	Activity	Sequence & Repetition	Coaching Points	Muscle Group	Fitness Component	Beg	Inter	Advan	Music
WARM UP	1, 2.3.	stretch. release into flat back swing 'ski' position.	repeat twice	posture:– long spine shoulders down tummy pulled in pelvis tucked under feet parallel.	whole body movement involves most muscle groups	mobility				slow tempo 4/4
A	5.6. 7.	curl around knees to roll up.	repeat once	back:– flat in the swing. rounded in in the roll up.		rhythmical loose and limbering stretch	*	all levels	*	red box by
no. 1-8	8.	stretch.	repeat whole A sequence twice	breath:– out on the swing – in rolling up						simply red

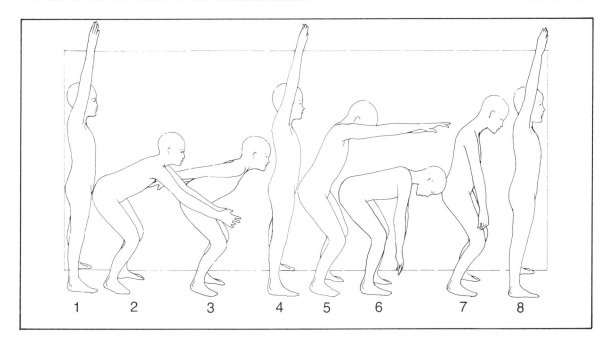

1   2   3   4   5   6   7   8

Sec	Fig no.	Activity	Sequence & Repetition	Coaching Points	Muscle Group	Fitness Component	Beg	Inter	Advan	Music
		reach away from centre to stretch		maintain good posture						slow tempo 4/4
	1.2.	high	repeat with right and left arm once in each direction		muscles of the scapulae	flexibility and		all		red
	3.4.	forward		extend the stretches to full limit.		stretch	*	levels	*	box
B	5.6.	side								
	7.8.	down	repeat sequence B once							
no. 1–8		return to centre after each stretch	repeat sequence A twice							simply red

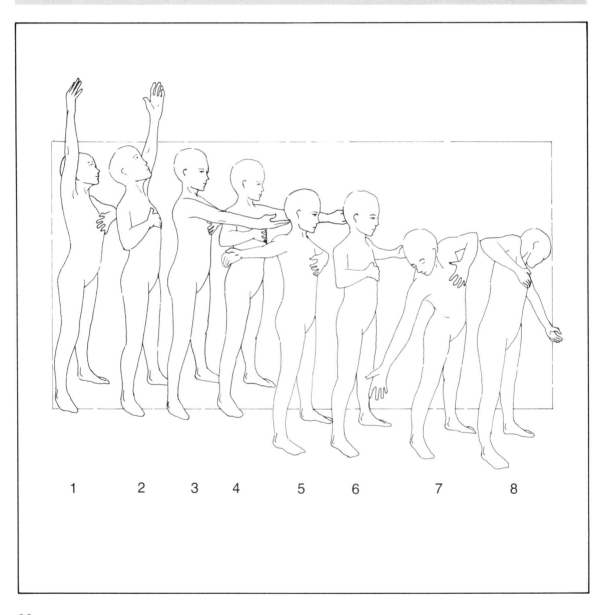

1 2 3 4 5 6 7 8

Sec	Fig no.	Activity	Sequence & Repetition	Coaching Points	Muscle Group	Fitness Component	Beg	Inter	Advan	Music
		stretches away from centre and back-allowing knees to bend	stretches on the right and left in each direction	alignment:– make sure that distribution of weight is correct-knee over toe when bending	muscles of the scapulea	flexibility				slow tempo 4/4
C	1.2. 3.4. 5.6. 7.8.		repeat 8 high over 8 forward and 8 side and 8 down		trapezius teres major latissimus dorsi		*	all levels	*	red box
no. 1–8			repeat sequence A twice repeat C again once repeat A twice		thigh muscles quadriceps	stretches				simply red

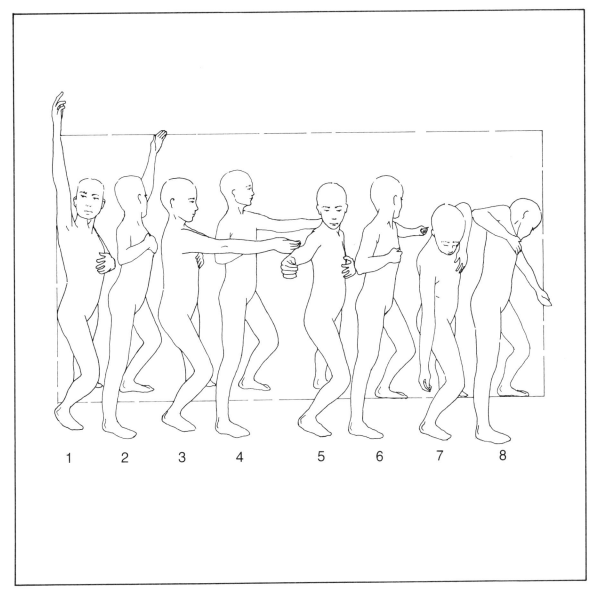

1   2   3   4   5   6   7   8

Sec	Fig no.	Activity	Sequence & Repetition	Coaching Points	Muscle Group	Fitness Component	Beg	Inter	Advan	Music
WARM UP SPEC	1.2.	nod head forward return to centre.	repeat once in each direction to the right and then to the left	lift the head elongating out of the spine	sternomastoid	posture				slow tempo 4/4
D	3.4.	tilt head to side return to centre.			splenius semispinalis-capitis	flexibility				red box
	5.6.	lift head up to look high return centre	repeat whole sequence twice.	keep the movement under control.			*	all levels	*	
no. 1–8	7.8.	turn to side and centre				stretch				simply red

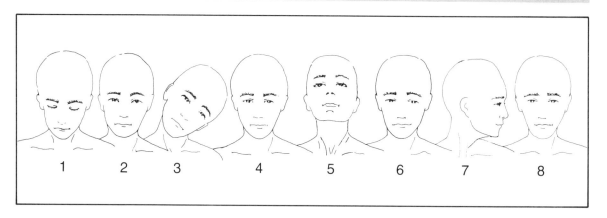

1   2   3   4   5   6   7   8

Sec	Fig no.	Activity	Sequence & Repetition	Coaching Points	Muscle Group	Fitness Component	Beg	Inter	Advan	Music
		gently rotate the head forward and lift out to the side turning to look.	repeat to the right and left	lengthen neck first	sternomastoid splenius	posture				slow tempo tempo 4/4
E					semispinalis-capitis	flexibility	*	all levels	*	red box
no. 1–7			repeat the sequence four times	rotate slowly with control.		stretch				simply red

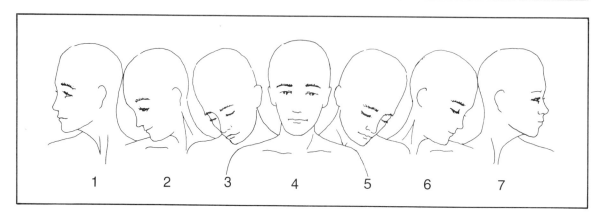

1   2   3   4   5   6   7

Sec	Fig no.	Activity	Sequence & Repetition	Coaching Points	Muscle Group	Fitness Component	Beg	Inter	Advan	Music
WARM UP	1.	stand with a relaxed knee		avoid locking out the knee joint	most of the muscles attached to the scapulae- upper back.	flexibility				fast tempo 4/4
	2.3.	gently circle	circle arms four							
	4.5.	the shoulders keeping a bent arm.	times	keep shoulders down and relaxed while circling.		mobility				
F	6.	from centre	to right three		obliques postural- muscles lying under the sacrospinalis	stretch	*	all levels	*	snake charmer
	7.8.	twist torso	return centre to left three	keep hips to the front 'square'.						
no. 1–8	9.	keeping arms bent.	return centre repeat sequence 3.							John Hiatt

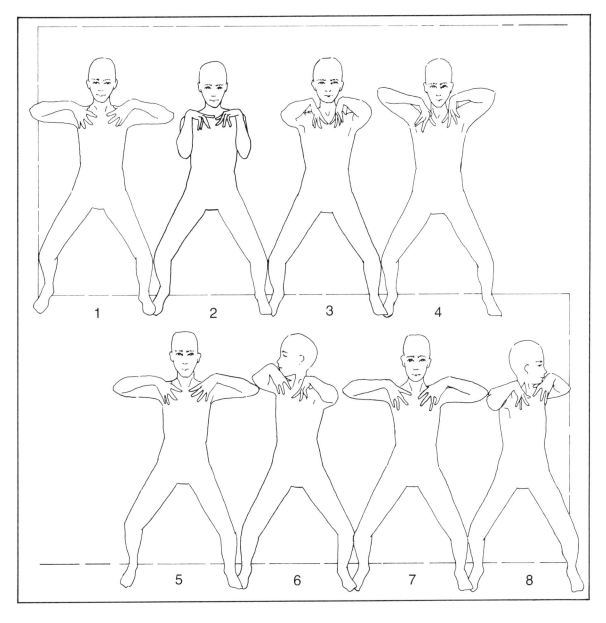

Sec	Fig no.	Activity	Sequence & Repetition	Coaching Points	Muscle Group	Fitness Component	Beg	Inter	Advan	Music
	1.	stand with a relaxed knee		keep weight balance forward.	muscles of the scapulae and upper back	flexibility	keep knees relaxed only	deeper knee bend	full plie	fast tempo
	2.3.	repeat arm								
	4.5.	circling. deepen the knee bend to curl forward round & up.	circle arms four times		quadriceps-gracilis adductor-magnus					snake charmer
G	6.7.	chest press		hold thighs open & pull up from knee joint into hip.		muscle strength				John Hiatt white nights
no. 1–9	8.	from high	press & release four times.		deltoid pectoralis major					
	9.	down to full plie & hold								

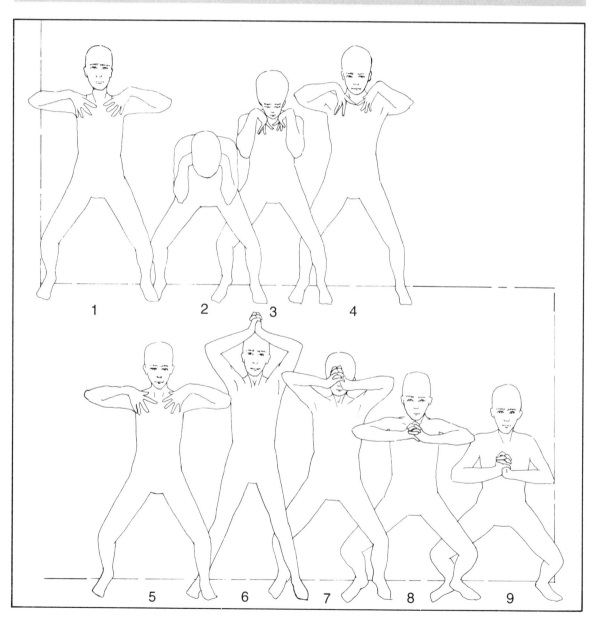

1   2   3   4

5   6   7   8   9

Sec	Fig no.	Activity	Sequence & Repetition	Coaching Points	Muscle Group	Fitness Component	Beg	Inter	Advan	Music
	1.	palms pressed together	repeat three twists to right	keep the hips square forward while torso twists	obliques postural muscles lying under the sacrospinalis	muscle strength	knees relaxed only	deeper knee bend	full plie	fast tempo
	2.	twist torso	return centre							
	3.	and return	three twists to left							
	4.	to centre	return. repeat twice	maintain posture		endurance				
H	5.6.	relax knees release arms	three twists to right & left once	keep thighs pulled open and up into hip.	deltoid pectoralis major					snake charmer
	7.8.	twist torso and return	twist right & left eight times.		quadriceps adductor	conditioning				
no. 1–8		to centre.			magnus gracilis					John Hiatt

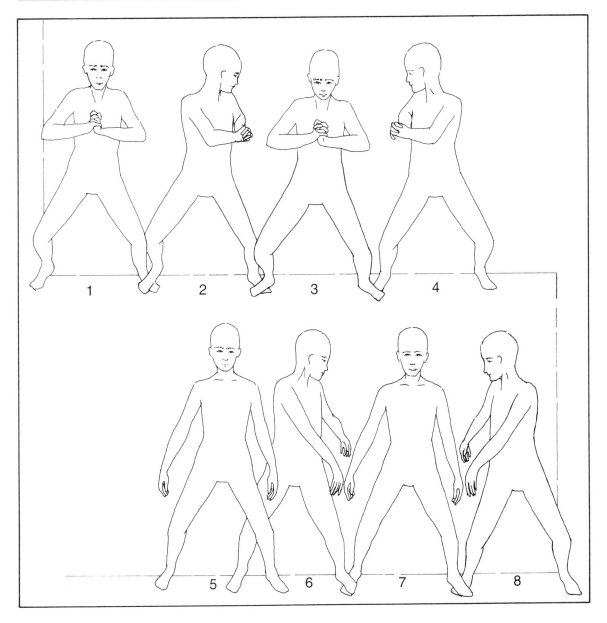

1   2   3   4

5   6   7   8

Sec	Fig no.	Activity	Sequence & Repetition	Coaching Points	Muscle Group	Fitness Component	Beg	Inter	Advan	Music
WARM UP	1.2.	reach out diagonally across body	repeat eight on right & left	with rapid changes of direction	muscles of upper & lower back.	flexibility	curl elbow to knee only.	deepen the curl to ankle for greater flexi-bility	deepen the curl to ankle for greater flexi-bility	fast tempo
	3.4.	bring level	repeat sixteen to right & left	keep weight forward and knee alignment correct.		mobility				
	5.6.	lower & curl arm into body (knee) (ankle)			thigh muscles	cardiovascular fitness				snake charmer
I	7.8.	curl	repeat right & left eight times		rectus abdom inus + action of r/l external and internal oblique working together in rotation					
no. 1–10	9.10.	& stretch								John Hiatt

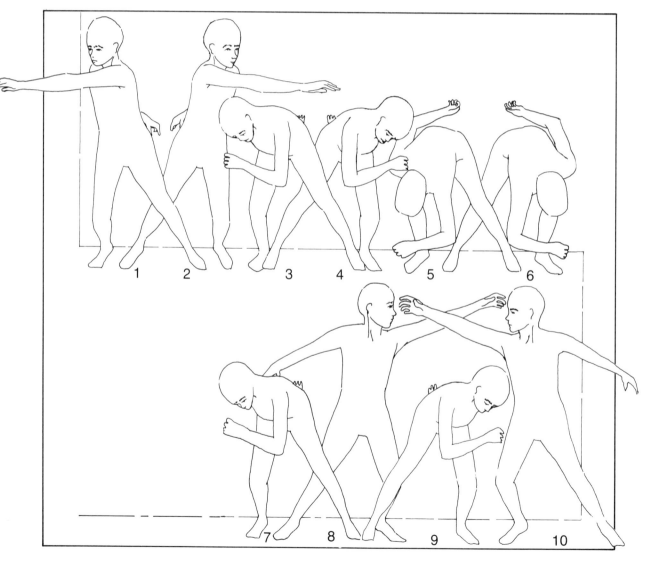

Sec	Fig no.	Activity	Sequence & Repetition	Coaching Points	Muscle Group	Fitness Component	Beg	Inter	Advan	Music
	1.3.	relaxed knee bends and swinging arms	repeat side bends four to right-relax	even weight distribution		flexibility				fast tempo
	2.4.	pull over into side bends. keep knees relaxed.	centre two swings four to left two centre swings repeat sequence four times	keep lateral flexion on a sideways plane avoid tipping forward or arching backward	oblique abdominals quadratis lumborum rectus abdom inus + action of r & l external and internal oblique working together in rotation	mobility stretch	*	all levels	*	snake charmer John Hiatt
J										
no. 1–4										

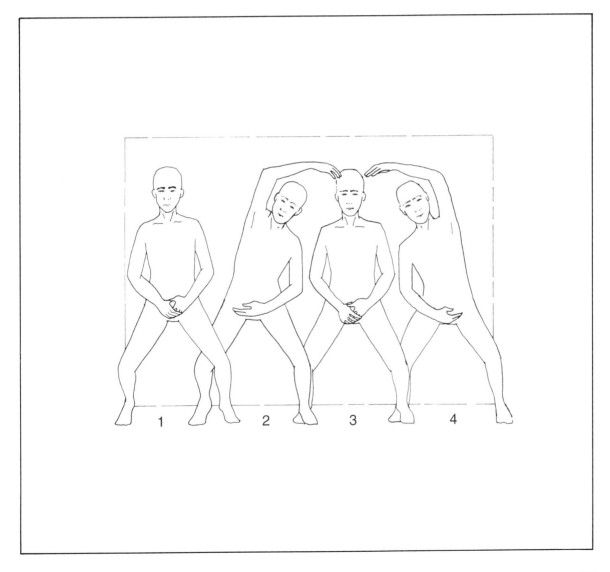

1   2   3   4

87

Sec	Fig no.	Activity	Sequence & Repetition	Coaching Points	Muscle Group	Fitness Component	Beg	Inter	Advan	Music
	1.	stretch high	two repetitions	avoid bending	muscles	stretch	drop as low		attempt	wrap
	2.	drop half	on a slow count	forward on the low	of upper and		as personal		to drop	hcr
		way hands		drop down	lower back		flexibility		to low	up
		clap thighs					allows		squat and	
	3.	sink low	sixteen repetitions	keep the feeling of					touch	
	4.	rise half way		squatting opening					floor	
		and clap		the thighs	thigh muscles	mobility				Elton
K										John
	5.9.	repeat with	sixteen repetitions			cardiovascular				fast
		high stretch	fast tempo			fitness				tempo
		to right and								
		left								
nos 1–9										

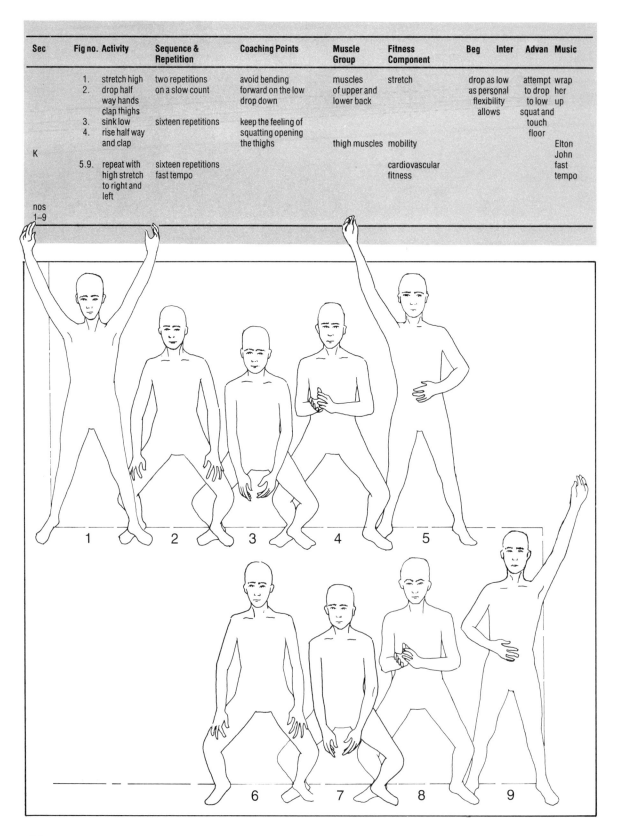

1 2 3 4 5

6 7 8 9

Sec	Fig no.	Activity	Sequence & Repetition	Coaching Points	Muscle Group	Fitness Component	Beg	Inter	Advan	Music
	1.2.	stretch and push heels high-return centre-bend knees and pulse at low level.	hold high stretch four beats. hold low position four beats.	do not allow the body to overbalance – or ankles to roll	lasissimus-dorsi deltoids trapezius	muscle endurance	hold as low as personal flexibility allows.	deepen to full plie	deepen to full plie	wrap her up Elton John
L	5.6.	raise right heel and lower-left heel and lower to low	four times slowly eight times faster	grip thighs pulling inward	quadriceps gastrocnemius soleus tibialis-anterior tibialis -posterior	stretch				
no. 1–8	7.8.	holding low position-push hips to right & left.	eight times.	release the low held position if the body bends forward.	hip abductors and adductors					

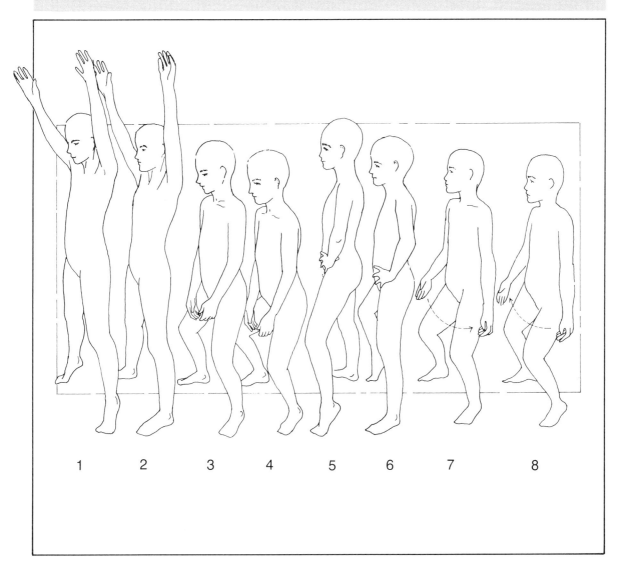

1   2   3   4   5   6   7   8

Sec	Fig no.	Activity	Sequence & Repetition	Coaching Points	Muscle Group	Fitness Component	Beg	Inter	Advan	Music
	1.2.	pelvic tilt & release back	repeat four times slowly.	relax knees from the low held position if the body tilts forward or ankles begin to roll outward		muscle endurance	hold only as low as pers-onal flexi-bility allows	deepen to full plie	deepen to full plie	wrap her up
M	3.4.	holding the low knees bent position raise both heels and lower.	repeat four times slowly.		quadriceps gastrocnemius soleus tibialis anterior/ posterior	stretch				
	5.6.	keeping knees bent– rotate hips to right	repeat twice to right.		rectus abdom inus and hip flexors and extensors.					Elton John
no. 1-8	7.8.	rotate to left. left.	repeat twice to left.							

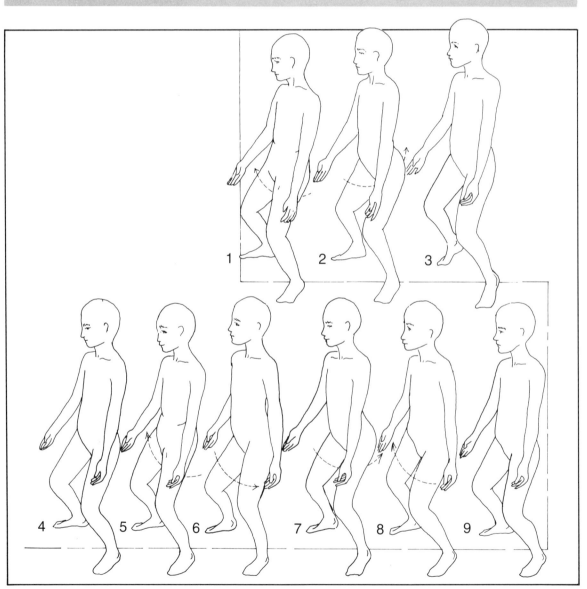

90

Sec	Fig no.	Activity	Sequence & Repetition	Coaching Points	Muscle Group	Fitness Component	Beg	Inter	Advan	Music
	1.	bending	take eight beats	approach the flat	quadriceps	flexibility	keep	extend the range		wrap
	2.3.	knees lower	to prepare position	back position very			bent	of movement as		her
		back with care		carefully through the			knee	fig. 4.5.		up
		lengthen	hold each position	bent knee– return to			position			
		forward flat	3.4.5. for eight	standing position in			through			
		back.	beats	same way			out			
N	4.5.	ease the		*hold* the flat back		stretch				Elton
		legs back		lengthening from top	abdominals					John
		straight		of head– look at floor	rectus abdom					
		lengthen			inus iliopsoas					
		arms wide								
	6.7.	relax knees	swing for eight			mobility				
		and arms	beats. repeat seq.							
no.		swing loosely	four times		hamstrings					
1–8	8.	roll up to	unroll for eight	do *not* bounce						
		straight	beats							

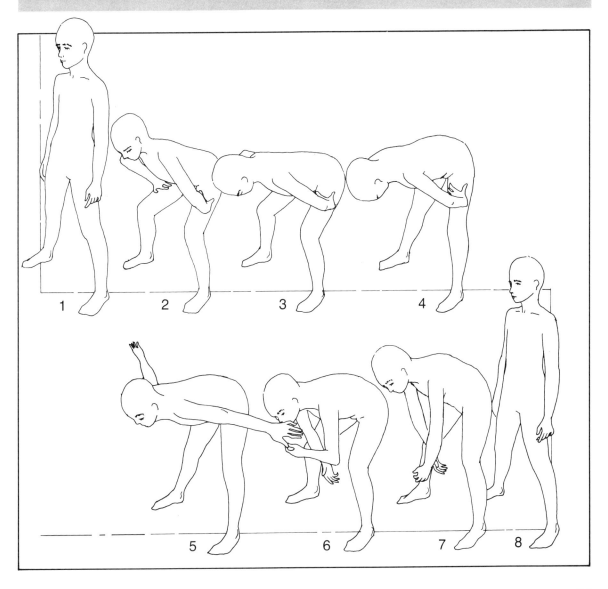

1   2   3   4

5   6   7   8

Sec	Fig no.	Activity	Sequence & Repetition	Coaching Points	Muscle Group	Fitness Component	Beg	Inter	Advan	Music
	1.2.	place feet together turned out. lower & rise	repeat slowly four times	hold the thighs out pulling up from knee into hip	quadriceps femoris	muscle endurance	release knees slightly to assist	deepen according to ability		wrap her up
	3.4.	holding low position pull up right and left heel	four times slowly eight times fast tempo		gastrocnemius soleus tibialis anterior/ posterior		good posture and balance			Elton John
0	5.6.	holding low position tilt hips to right and left	repeat eight times fast tempo	keep torso erect holding posture						
no. 1–8	7.8.	holding low position pelvic tilt forward and release back	repeat four times slowly		gluteals a combination of hip flexors and extensors abductors and adductors	stretch				

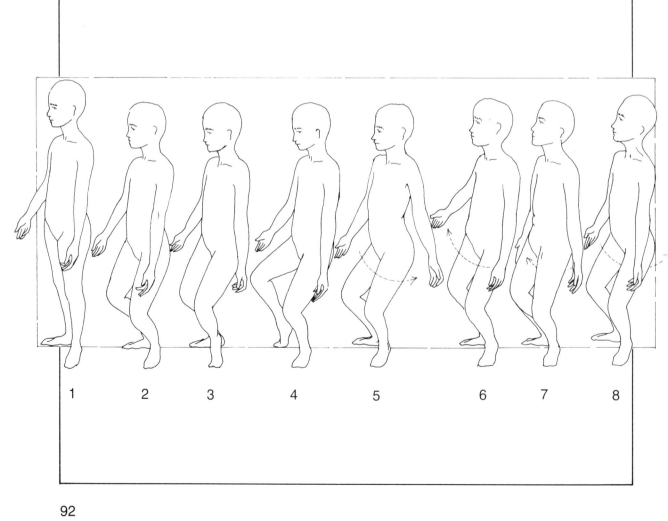

1   2   3   4   5   6   7   8

Sec	Fig no.	Activity	Sequence & Repetition	Coaching Points	Muscle Group	Fitness Component	Beg	Inter	Advan	Music
P	1.2.	raise both heels and lower with knees held in low bent position	repeat four times slowly	relax knees slightly if body finds difficulty in balancing	quadriceps femoris gastrocnemius soleus tibialis anterior/ posterior	muscle endurance	release knees slightly to assist good posture and balance	deepen according to ability		wrap her up
	3.4.	rotate hips	repeat twice to		gluteals	stretch				Elton John
No. 1-7	5.6. 7.	to right and left	the right and twice to the left		abdominals erector spinae					

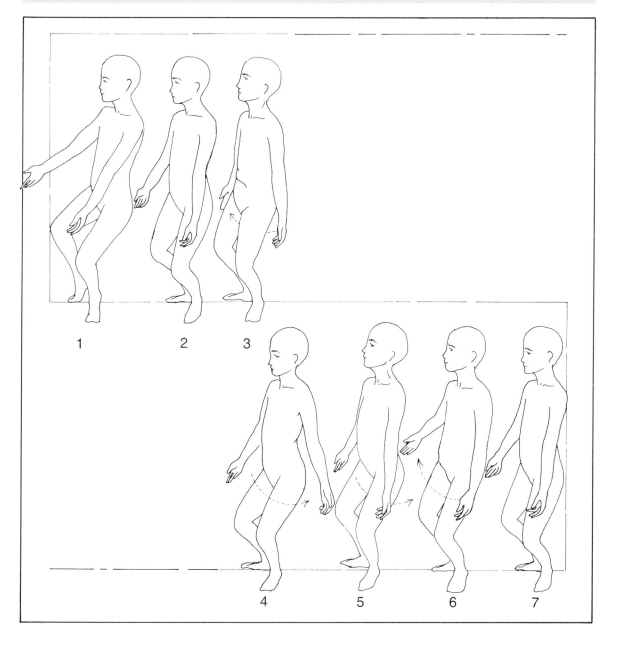

1 2 3

4 5 6 7

Sec	Fig no.	Activity	Sequence & Repetition	Coaching Points	Muscle Group	Fitness Component	Beg	Inter	Advan	Music
	1.2.	place feet in narrow parallel lower & rise	repeat four times slowly	hold upper torso erect	quadriceps femoris	muscle endurance	release knees slightly	deepen according to ability		wrap her up
Q	3.4.	hold low position and pull up right & left heel.	repeat four times slowly eight times fast tempo	keep tail tucked under	gastrocnemius soleus tibialis anterior/ posterior		to assist good posture and balance			
	5.6.	holding low position tilt hips to right and left		maintain the parallel positions of thighs		stretch				
nos. 1–8	7.8.	holding low position pelvic tilt forward & back	repeat four times slowly		hip flexors and extensors					Elton John

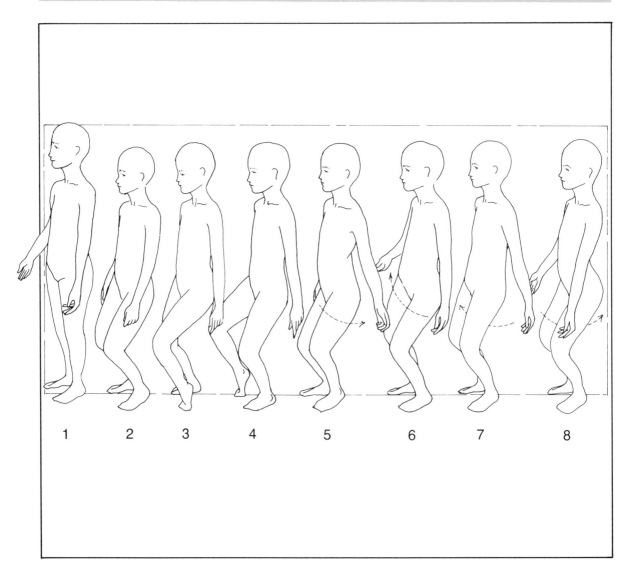

1 2 3 4 5 6 7 8

Sec	Fig no.	Activity	Sequence & Repetition	Coaching Points	Muscle Group	Fitness Component	Beg	Inter	Advan	Music
	1.2.	raise both heels and lower with knees held in low bent position	repeat four times slowly	relax knees slightly if body finds difficulty in balancing	quadriceps femoris gastrocnemius soleus tibialis anterior/	muscle endurance	release knees slightly good posture	deepen according to ability		wrap her up
R					posterior	stretch	and balance			Elton John
	3.4. 5.6. 7.	rotate hips to right and left	repeat twice to the right and twice to the left		gluteals abdominals erector spinae					
nos. 1-7										

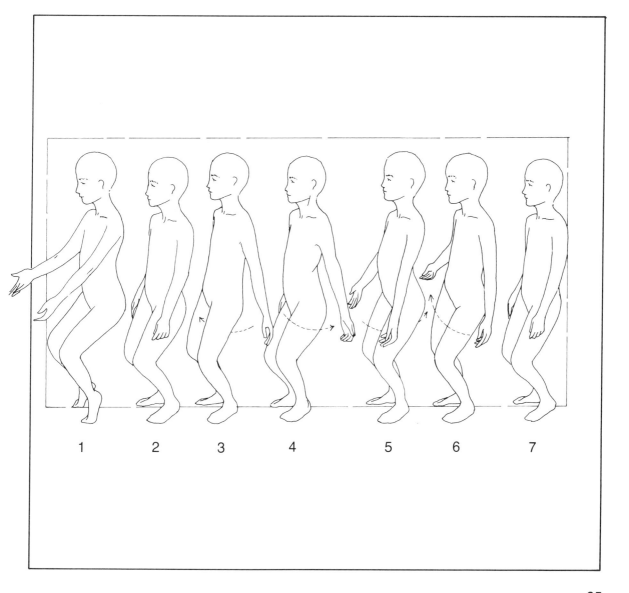

1   2   3   4   5   6   7

Sec	Fig no.	Activity	Sequence & Repetition	Coaching Points	Muscle Group	Fitness Component	Beg	Inter	Advan	Music
	1.3.	arms forward step forward in deep lunge keeping forward heel down. Stretch back leg pressing heel to floor	repeat sixteen times arms forward sixteen times arms high	1. correct alignment of knee over toe 2. press heel down in gentle sustained stretch not jerky	hamstrings	flexibility				wrap her up
S	2.4.	bring arms to high and continue the stretch	on right foot and left foot		achilles tendon	stretch	*	all levels	*	Elton John
no. 1–4										

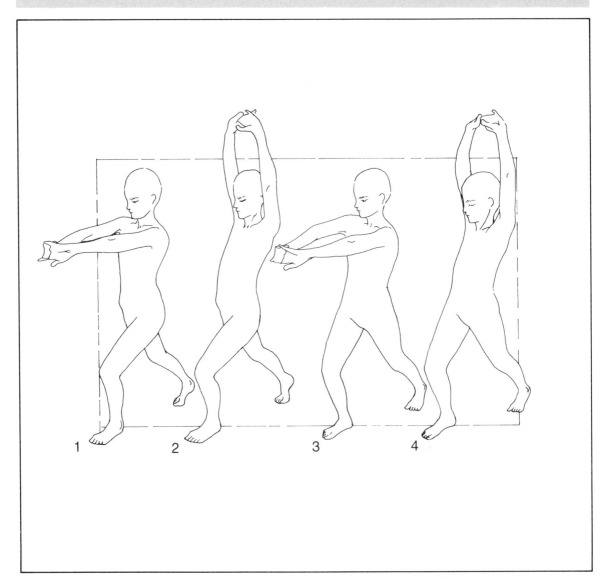

1   2   3   4

Aerobic Section 20 minutes continuous movement activity.

Sec	Fig no.	Activity	Sequence & Repetition	Coaching Points	Muscle Group	Fitness Component	Beg	Inter	Advan	Music
a e r . o b i c	1.2.	calf raises push heels high and lower	repeat slowly sixteen times	squeeze inner thighs together to hold high balance and avoid rolling ankles	gastrocnemius soleus	muscle strength				money for nothing
	3.4. 5.	from high balance lower one heel at a time	repeat slowly eight times double time sixteen repetitions		tibialis anterior posterior	stretch	*	all levels	*	
A no. 1–10	6.7. 8.	peel the foot off the floor heel/ball/toe	slowly eight times	feel the parts of the foot through the stretch						
	9.10.	release back to floor ball/heel/toe	double time sixteen repetitions							Dire Straits

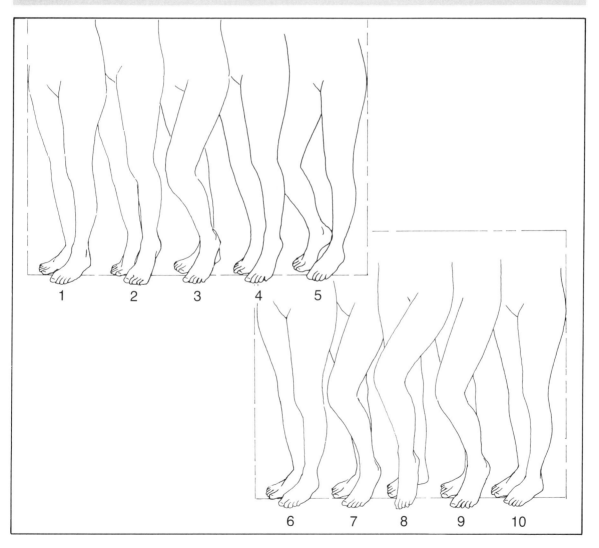

1   2   3   4   5

6   7   8   9   10

97

Sec	Fig no.	Activity	Sequence & Repetition	Coaching Points	Muscle Group	Fitness Component	Beg	Inter	Advan	Music
	1.2.	peel the foot as before to lift just off floor	eight times slowly sixteen doubletime	encourage good plantar flexion stretching toe hard	tibialis anterior	stretch				money for nothing
B	3.4.	release back to floor-toe/ ball/heel								
	5.6.	peel foot as before to lift higher			quadriceps	muscle strength				
	7.8.	release back to floor toe/ball/heel	eight times slowly sixteen double time		iliopsoas		*	all levels	*	
no. 1-8										Dire Straits

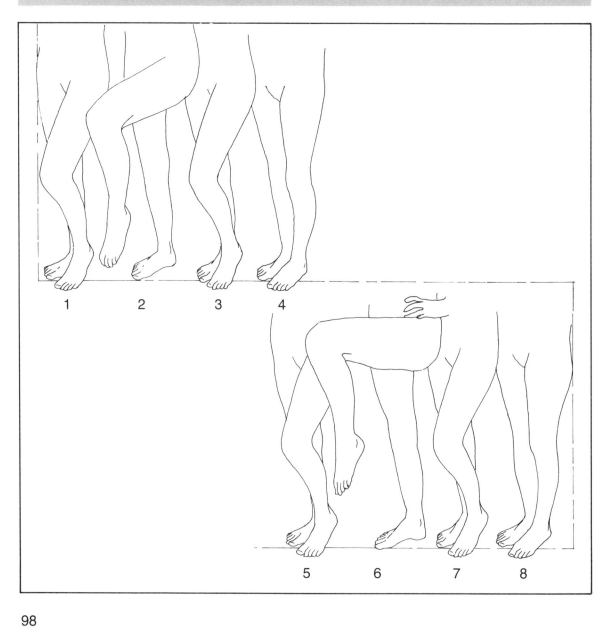

1   2   3   4

5   6   7   8

Sec	Fig no.	Activity	Sequence & Repetition	Coaching Points	Muscle Group	Fitness Component	Beg	Inter	Advan	Music
	1.2. 3.	Peel the foot off floor – open thigh point toe	8 times slowly then 16 times fast	Encourage resilience in the ankle. Release the heel back into floor, on landing to prevent jarring.	Tibialis anterior	Stretch	As Fig I.2 3	As Fig 4.5	As Fig 6.7	Money for Nothing
CI	4.5.	Repeat as above, rising on the support leg-ball foot	8 times fast		Quadriceps	Muscle strength				
	6.7.	repeat with spring off floor.	8 times fast		Iliopsoas	Cardiovascular endurance				
no. 1–7										

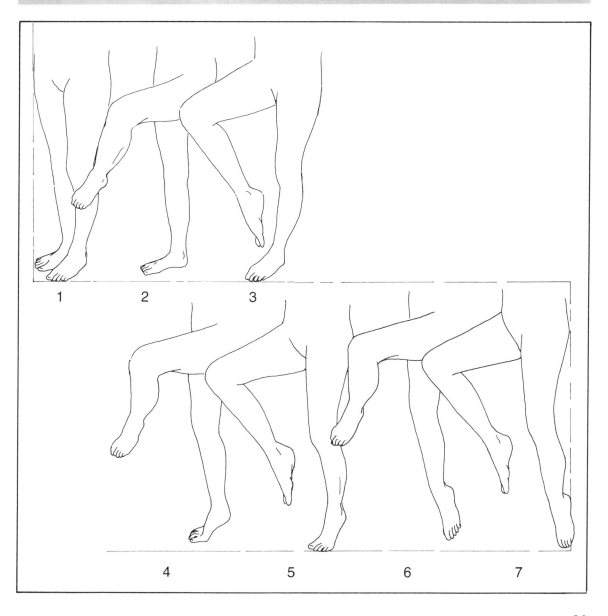

1   2   3

4   5   6   7

Sec	Fig no.	Activity	Sequence & Repetition	Coaching Points	Muscle Group	Fitness Component	Beg	Inter	Advan	Music
C2	1.2 3.4. 5 8	Walk forward and lift leg pointing toe	Repeat 4 sequences forward & back	Make sure the group is well spaced	Tibialis anterior	Muscle strength	As Fig. 1.2.3	As Fig. 4.5	As Fig. 6.7	Money for Nothing
No. 1–8			Variations can be made by repeating the forward and back sequence, turning in a square to the right.	Practice forward and back without the leg lifting at first. Practice turning in a square before adding the leg lift on the turn.	Quadriceps Iliopsoas	Cardiovascular Fitness				
			Repeat 4 sequences							

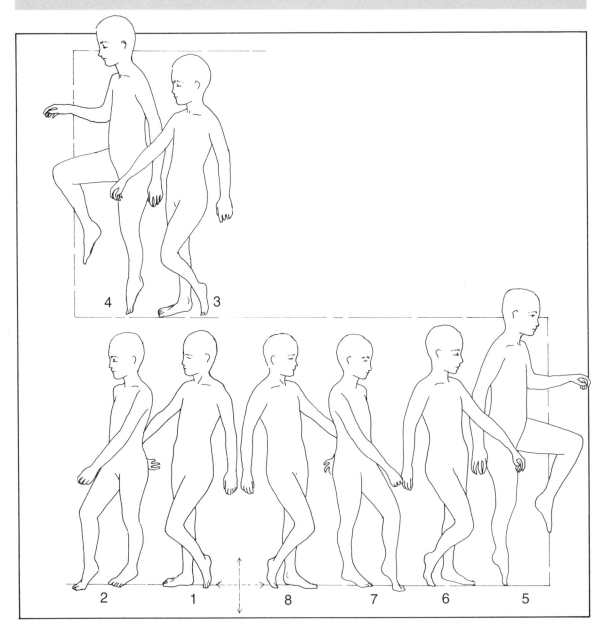

Sec	Fig no.	Activity	Sequence & Repetition	Coaching Points	Muscle Group	Fitness Component	Beg	Inter	Advan	Music
D		Variation on previous footwork stretching legs forward with a lift.	Repeat 16 times Repeat 4 sequences	Build up new ideas gradually	Muscles of lower limb & upper shoulder area	Muscle strength & endurance	Keep one foot in contact with the floor through out.	Raise heel higher lifting on ball of foot	Small spring off floor	As above
No.										
1—8		Travelling step with a spring. Raise & lower arms 'Sailor's Hornpipe' arms.	forward & back Turn in a square	Establish the foot work, before adding arms & multi-dimensional travel. Encourage breathing Coach resilient feet and ankles.		Cardiovascular fitness				

1   2   3   4   5   6   7   8

Sec	Fig no.	Activity	Sequence & Repetition	Coaching Points	Muscle Group	Fitness Component	Beg	Inter	Advan	Music
E	1.2	Footwork heel & toe	Repeat on right and left side –	Encourage positive flexion of the foot stretching hard on to heel & toe.	Tibialis anterior	Muscle strength	Keep Reps simple	Increase up to working	Reps 4 times one leg	As Above
	3.4	Plantar Dorsi flexion	up to 4 each side. Repeat turning in a square to R & L.		Tibialis posterior	Stretch				
No 1.6	5.6	Release leg muscles shaking loose on each side	As above.	Make sure heel drops on to floor on working foot. Allow calf to relax in shaking leg.		Cardiovascular fitness	Release more often	Add multi-dimen-sional work.	square	

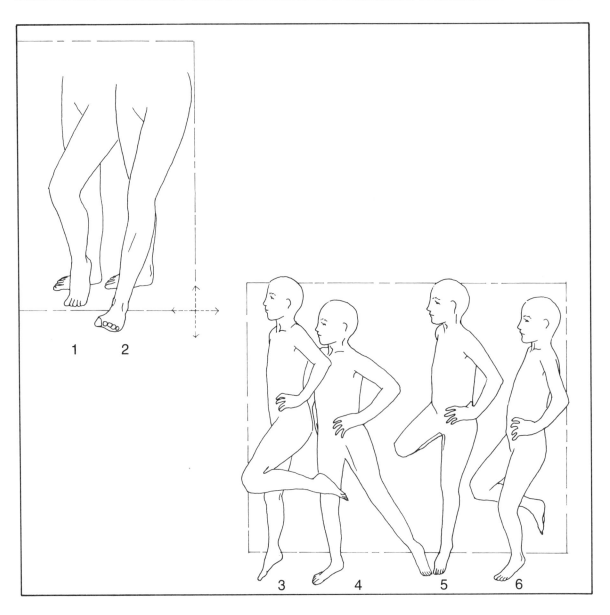

1   2

3   4   5   6

Sec	Fig no.	Activity	Sequence & Repetition	Coaching Points	Muscle Group	Fitness Component	Beg	Inter	Advan	Music
F	1.2.	Low level springy walk continuously stretch arms high alternate	– throughout Take 4 beats to stretch then 2 beats	1. Establish good body carriage and full stretch through the feet – lifting the body upward	Muscles of upper shoulder area, and lower limb.	Muscle endurance				Fast Tempo
No. 1-6	3.4.	arms to side		2. Encourage breathing		Cardiovascular fitness	Low Drop the arms if tired	impact	footwork	What you get is what you see.
	5.6.	Both arms high side	– slowly at first then fast.	3. Add variations in arm work gradually.						Tina Turner

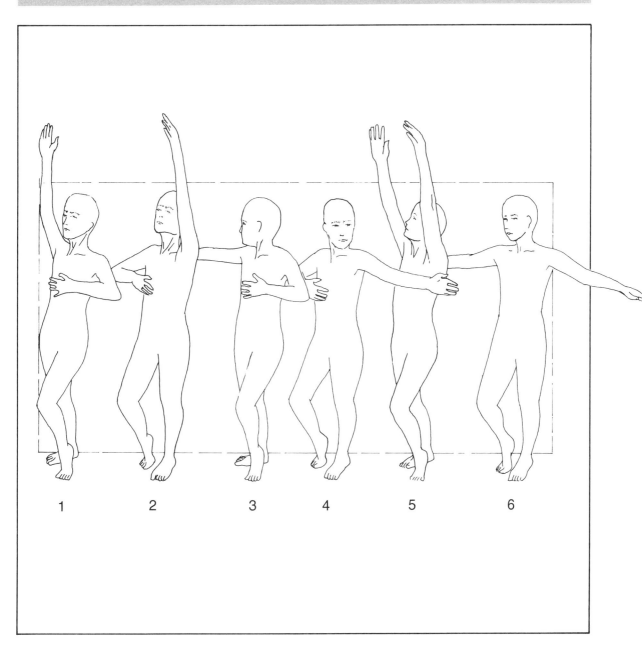

1   2   3   4   5   6

Sec	Fig no.	Activity	Sequence & Repetition	Coaching Points	Muscle Group	Fitness Component	Beg	Inter	Advan	Music
		Low level continuous springy walk	– throughout	1. Keep shoulders down & relaxed	Muscles of lower limb	Mobility				As above
G	1.2	Flexion & extension of wrist.	16 repetitions	2. Try not to 'lockout' the elbows.	Hip shoulder area	Cardiovascular fitness	Less Reps	Build up	the reps	
No.							More relaxed			
1–5	3.4	Add forward & backward circling.	16 repetitions each direction	Keep circles small	Biceps Supinators Pronators		swings			
	5.	Relaxed swings to release tension.	8 repetitions							

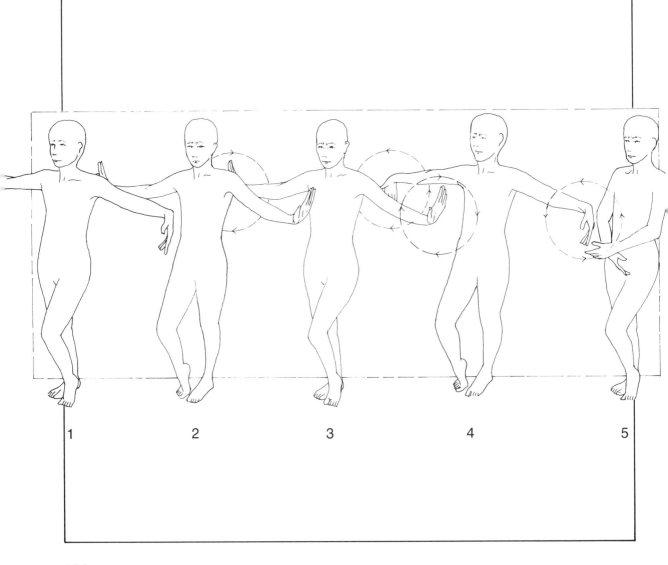

1   2   3   4   5

Sec	Fig no.	Activity	Sequence & Repetition	Coaching Points	Muscle Group	Fitness Component	Beg	Inter	Advan	Music
		Low level continuous springy walk	– throughout		Muscles of lower limb	Mobility				As above
H	1.2 3.4.	Raise arms in circle upward squeezing & stretching fingers.	16 counts to high 16 counts to low	Work fingers strongly	Hip Shoulder area	Cardiovascular fitness		Raise arms to increase to medium high level only.		
No 1–5	5	Repeat lower the arms to stretch down.	Repeat 4 sequences		Biceps Supinator Pronator					

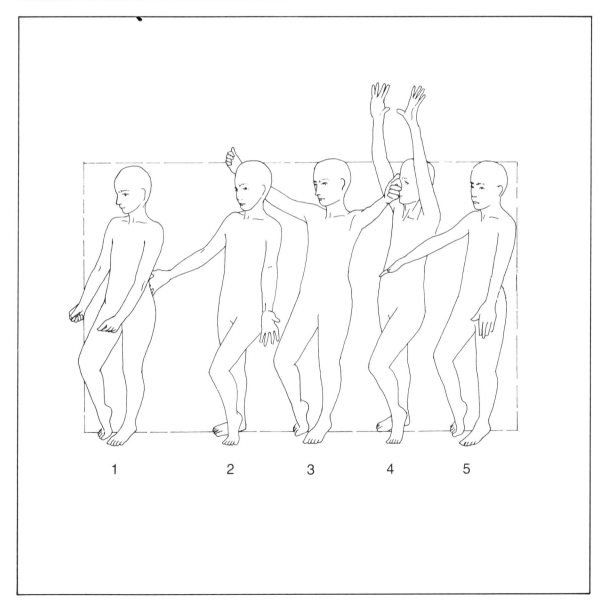

1   2   3   4   5

Sec	Fig no.	Activity	Sequence & Repetition	Coaching Points	Muscle Group	Fitness Component	Beg	Inter	Advan	Music
		Low level continuous springy walk	– throughout							As above
I	1.2. 3.	Scissor the arms in front Raise up & down	8 reps in front. 8 up 8 down	1. Avoid 'locking out' elbow joint. 2. Relax shoulders in in the upward stretch	Muscles of lower limb Hip	Muscle endurance	Only 'scissor' forward Not up	build up	higher	levels
No 1–8	4.5 6	'Scissor' in front of hips & open wide.	2 reps in front & hold open	3. Keep the last movement relaxed.	Shoulder area	Cardiovascular fitness	More rest swings			
	6.7. 8.	'Scissor' behind & open wide	2 reps behind & hold open		Forearm Triceps Anconeus					

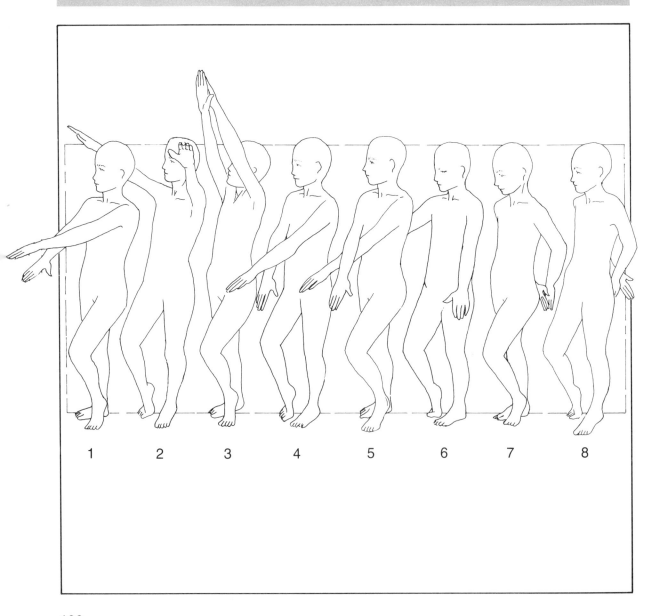

1   2   3   4   5   6   7   8

Sec	Fig no.	Activity	Sequence & Repetition	Coaching Points	Muscle Group	Fitness Component	Beg	Inter	Advan	Music
		Shows 3 levels of movement activity.	Repeat each style of movement through with the class to demonstrate how it feels.	1. Emphasize that heels must release down into the floor, at each level of movement – keep ankle resilient	Muscles of lower back					Fast Tempo
J	1.2	Low level springy walk pushing up off heel & release			Hip	Cardiovascular fitness	As Nos 1.2	As Nos 3.4	As Nos 5.6	Holding out for a Hero
No. 1–6	3.4	Toes just leave floor-heel release down.		2. Encourage good body carriage, safe alignment of lower limbs.	Lower limb.					
	5.6.	High level jog Heels kick up toward bottom and release down.		3. Encourage and monitor breathing.						Bonnie Tyler

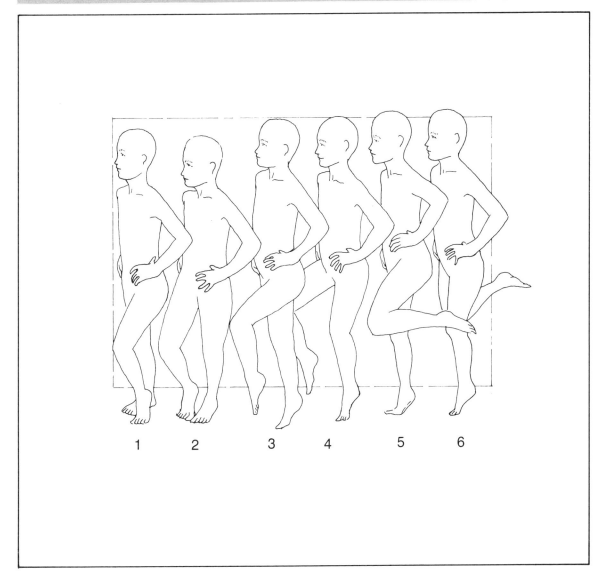

1 2 3 4 5 6

Sec	Fig no.	Activity	Sequence & Repetition	Coaching Points	Muscle Group	Fitness Component	Beg	Inter	Advan	Music
		Lift feet alternately to side – touch ankle. Low level feet.	Repeat 4 on R. 4 on L. 4 sequences	1. Encourage good body posture – lift leg rather than bend body down.	As above		As Nos. 1.2	Prog- ress to Nos 3.4	Prog- ress to Nos 5.6	As Above
K No. 1–6	1.2 3.4	As above – 2 lifts each side	As above.	2. Keep ankle resilient Relax heel into floor	Gluteus medius minimus Tensor fascia latae	Cardiovascular fitness				
	5.6.	As above – 1 each side.	4 sequences.							

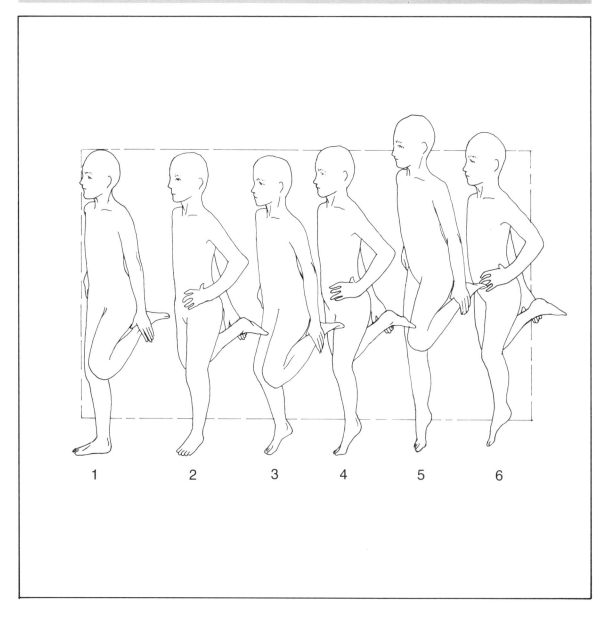

1   2   3   4   5   6

Sec	Fig no.	Activity	Sequence & Repetition	Coaching Points	Muscle Group	Fitness Component	Beg	Inter	Advan	Music
	1.2	Lift feet alternately behind body to touch opposite hand.	The number of repetitions can be adjusted to suit the class fitness level.	1. Encourage good body carriage, lifting body up out of floor, not bending too much toward the lifting leg, or straining forward.	Iliopsoas Quadriceps Erector spinae	Muscle endurance	Low level foot-work	Prog-ress to springy heel	Foot leaving floor	As Above
L	3.4	As above but lift knee in front.								
No.	5.6	Lift knee to opposite elbow	Each activity can be mixed with low level walk to give relaxation & build up slowly.	2. Keep heel coming back down to floor, ankle resilient.	Biceps	Cardiovascular fitness				
1–10	7.8	Repeat with hands behind ears.								
	9.10	Add leg kick forward								

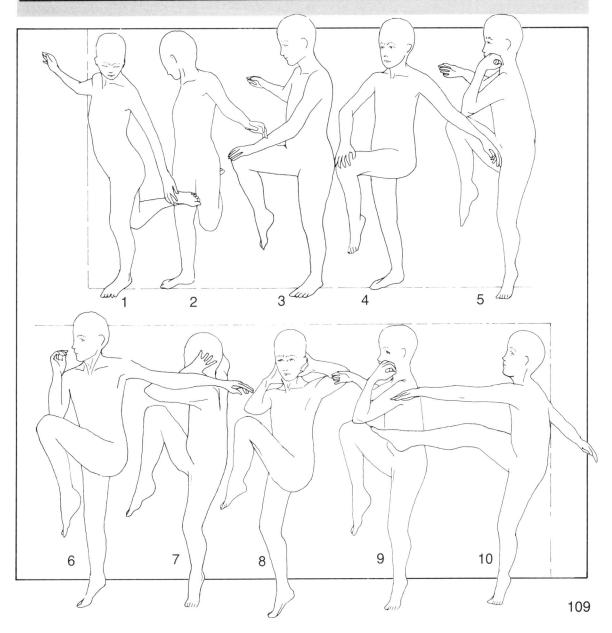

1   2   3   4   5

6   7   8   9   10

Sec	Fig no.	Activity	Sequence & Repetition	Coaching Points	Muscle Group	Fitness Component	Beg	Inter	Advan	Music
M No. 1–4	1.2 3.4.	Swivel the hips, lifting heels from floor-pulling body up and across. Repeat activity back to change direction.	Repeat from side to side continuously.	1. Keep the feet parallel as they lift and place down. 2. Keep foot movement strong springy and resilient.	Combined muscles of Hip Lower limb Feet & ankle	Cardiovascular fitness	Toes in touch with floor through-out Concen-trate on feet keeping parallel	Spring-ier heel lift	Just off floor	As above

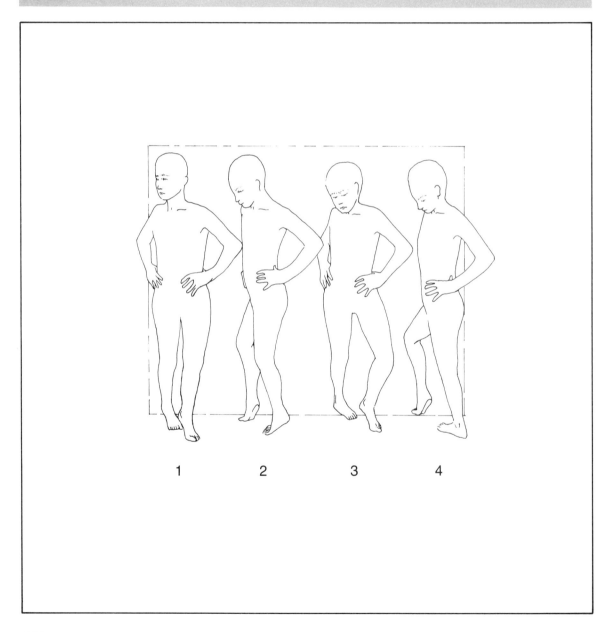

1   2   3   4

Sec	Fig no.	Activity	Sequence & Repetition	Coaching Points	Muscle Group	Fitness Component	Beg	Inter	Advan	Music
N	1.2 3.4	Pull in & reach high & wide.	On R side – 8 sequences On L side	Fig. 1.2.3.4. are quite strenuous if the approach vigorous						
No.	5.6 7.8	Pull in and spring out symmetrically punching alternate arms	– Repeat 4 times	Pull body weight low into centre each time to regain balance.	Most major muscle groups	Cardiovascular fitness	Nos. 1.2.3.4	Nos. 5.6.7.8	Nos. 9.10	As above
1–10	9.10	Pull in an spring out both arms high & wide.	– Repeat 4 times	Keep ankles resilient						

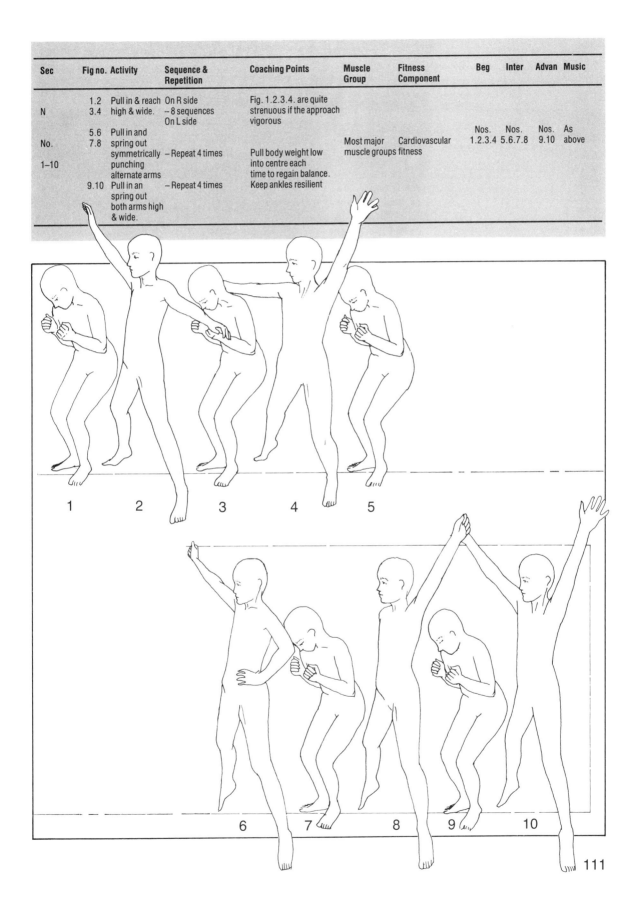

1   2   3   4   5

6   7   8   9   10

Take pulse for Target Zone monitoring: Warm down:

Sec	Fig no.	Activity	Sequence & Repetition	Coaching Points	Muscle Group	Fitness Component	Beg	Inter	Advan	Music
WARM DOWN	1.2	Bending from side to side swinging arms	Repeat 8 times.	Encourage continuation of movement activity	Obliques		– All	levels	–	Medium Tempo
A	3.4.	Maintaining knee bends	Repeat 16 times	Knees bending to warm down gradually	Biceps Triceps	Stretching				Don't waste my time
No.		Fold arms in to chest and stretch wide.		Encourage deep breathing to aid relaxation and recovery	Quadriceps Hamstrings					
1–7	5.6	Lunge forward in deep knee bend and lift up	Repeat 4 times							Whitney Houston
			Repeat 8 times							
	7	Lift half way								

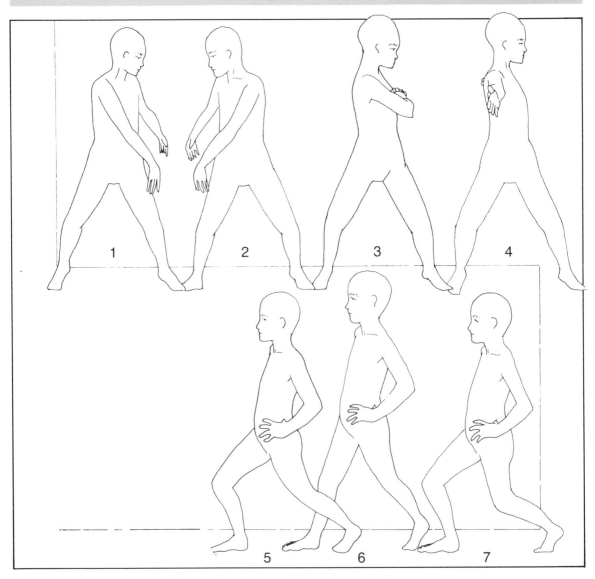

Sec	Fig no.	Activity	Sequence & Repetition	Coaching Points	Muscle Group	Fitness Component	Beg	Inter	Advan	Music
B	1.2 3	Bend knees and lower trunk forward bend & stretch slowly from side to side	– repeat 16 times	1. Keep feet parallel 2. Relax chest over thigh.	Rectus abdominus. Obliques	Stretch	Body only as low as mobility permits	As low as flexibility allows		As above
No										
1–7	4.5	Hold on one side and gently stretch the bent leg – add an arm	– Repeat 4 on R 4 on L. 4 sequences	3. Avoid 'locking out' knee in full stretch.	Quadriceps Hamstrings Gracilis		and also stretch only as far as is possible	– similarly with		stretches
	6.7	Bend knees unroll body	– Once to recover							

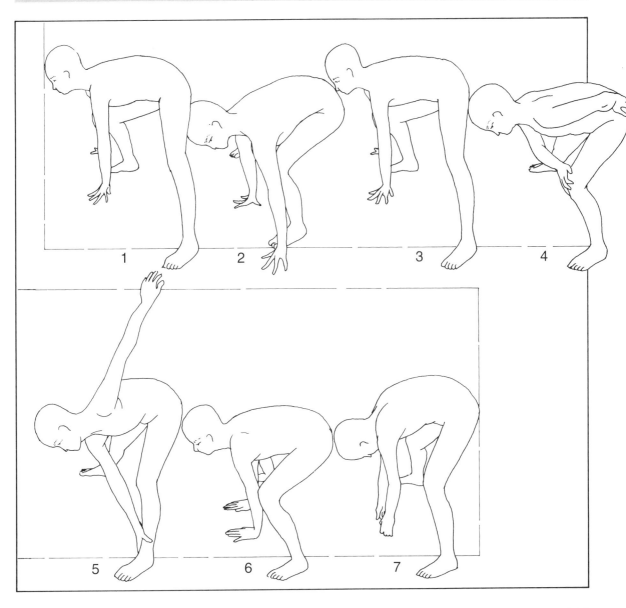

1   2   3   4

5   6   7

113

Sec	Fig no.	Activity	Sequence & Repetition	Coaching Points	Muscle Group	Fitness Component	Beg	Inter	Advan	Music
	1	Recover posture.	Hold 8 counts							As above
C.	2.3	Lunge each side	– Repeat 8 times	1. Keep correct alignment of knee over toe in lunge.	Quadriceps Gracilis	Stretch	Only go as low as flexi-	– Progress to		lower level
No.	4.5.	Bring body to lower level Press elbow inside thigh	– Repeat 8 times.	2. Make sure thigh and ankle do not roll inward at lower level	Hamstrings		bility allows			
1–9	6.7.	Long low lunge forward on one leg, stretch other leg.	– Repeat 16 times each leg.	3. Keep weight at back – forward bend of leg at 90° – lengthen backward.						
	8.9	Alternate legs;								

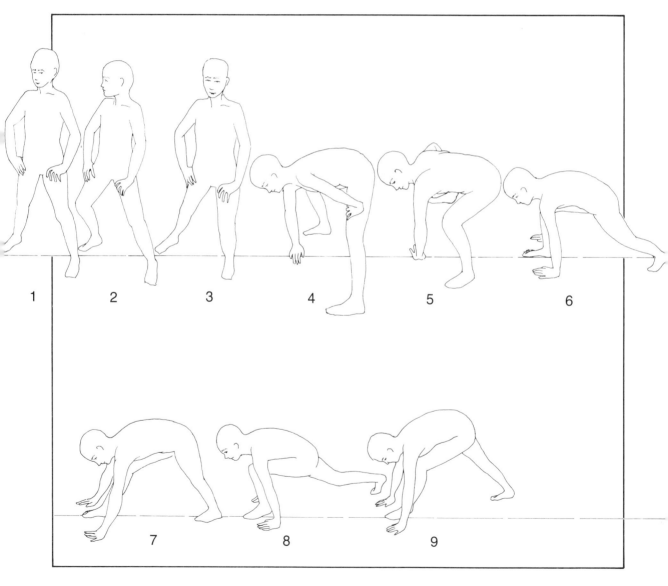

1

2

3

4

5

6

7

8

9

Sec	Fig no.	Activity	Sequence & Repetition	Coaching Points	Muscle Group	Fitness Component	Beg	Inter	Advan	Music
D	1.2.	Stretch alternate	– Repeat 8 R side 8 L side.		Hamstrings					
	3.	heels to floor then each heel in turn.	– 16 times	Slow stretches No bouncing		Stretch	– All	levels	–	As above
No. 1–6	4.5	Lower to long stretch of spine	– 16 counts	Relax head and shoulders	Quadratus lumborum Sacrospinalis					
	6	Relax prone and relax legs	– 16 counts.	Floppy legs.						

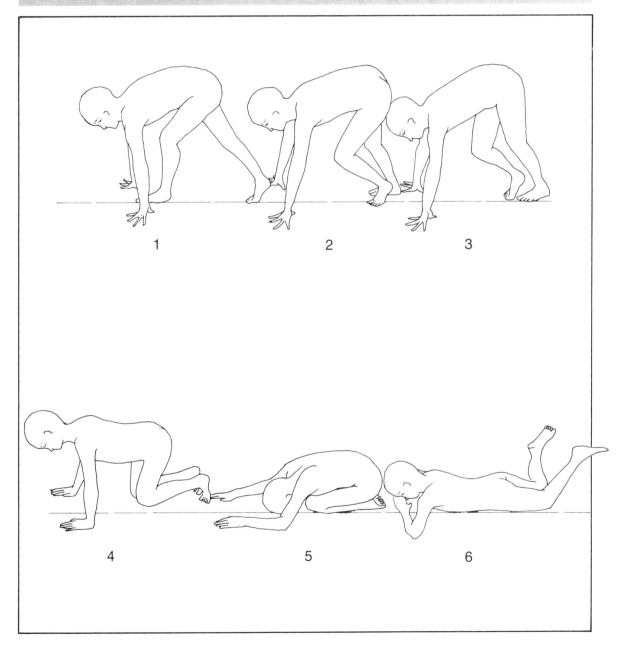

1

2

3

4

5

6

Sec	Fig no.	Activity	Sequence & Repetition	Coaching Points	Muscle Group	Fitness Component	Beg	Inter	Advan	Music
E	1.2.	Gentle spinal stretch and release	Take 4 counts to push and 4 to lower. Repeat 4 times.	2. Keep hips on floor Avoid over-arching.	Rectus abdominus Obliques	Stretch	Half-bend knees not full	– Full	knee	bend – As above
No. 1–6	3.4.	Pulse gently knees bent	– 8 counts	4. Keep weight forward pushing from hands.	Quatratus lumborum					
	5.6	Unroll slowly and stretch.	– 8 counts.	6. Relax torso into thighs breathing out	Sacrospinalis Quadriceps					

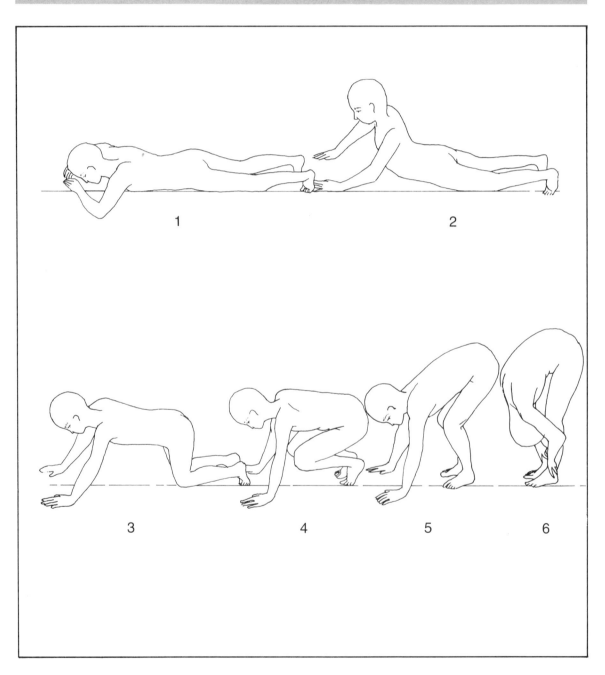

1

2

3

4

5

6

Sec	Fig no.	Activity	Sequence & Repetition	Coaching Points	Muscle Group	Fitness Component	Beg	Inter	Advan	Music
A BODY COND-ITION No. 1–8	1.2 3.4	Abduction of upper leg; Raising & lowering.	Repeat 8 times release	1. Maintain body alignment on side. Hips forward, torso lifted.	Abductors Tensor fascia latae and Gluteals	Muscle endurance	Less Reps:	– Inc	reps –	Baby's coming back
	5.6 7.8	Leg at right angles forward Raise & lower	Repeat 8 times	2. Squeeze buttock to assist leg lift. 3. Breathe out on the lift.						Eurythmics

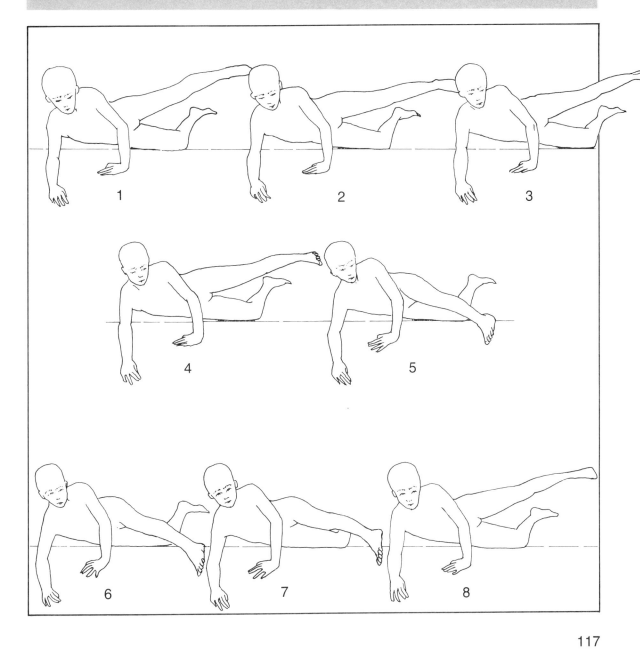

Sec	Fig no.	Activity	Sequence & Repetition	Coaching Points	Muscle Group	Fitness Component	Beg	Inter	Advan	Music
B	1.2.	From forward Bend knee in straighten out & lift	– 8 counts to complete sequence	1. Maintain side position.	Abductors Tensor fascia	Muscle endurance	Less Reps:	– Inc	Reps –	As above
	3.4	Repeat back		2. Avoid rolling backward on to buttock	latae					
	5.6.	& lift forward.	Repeat sequence 4 times	3. Raise leg only as high as hip allows.	Gluteals					
No. 1–10	7.8	Raise & lower leg toe in plantar flexion and dorsi-flexion.	8 times each leg	4. Keep torso low avoid arching back.	Hamstrings.					
	9									
	10.	Little lifts just above the floor.	16 counts each leg	Slow action is more effective, than fast.	Quadriceps					

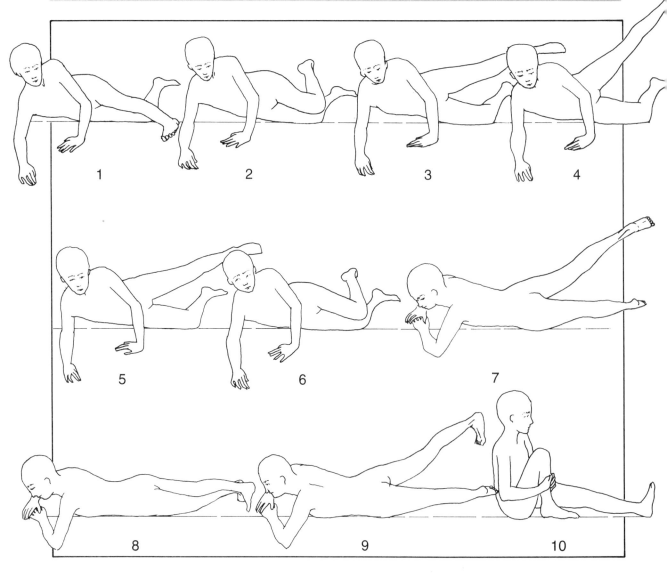

1 2 3 4

5 6 7

8 9 10

Sec	Fig no.	Activity	Sequence & Repetition	Coaching Points	Muscle Group	Fitness Component	Beg	Inter	Advan	Music
	1.2	Thigh Stretch	8 times each leg. leg.	1. Rest head on arm avoid arching back.	Quadriceps	Stretch	– All	levels –	Increase stretch by sqeez-	Money's too tight to mention
C No.	3.4. 5	From all fours stretch arm & leg; return to floor.	4 times each side	2. Keep movement slow & smooth. Keep horizontal line of body and hold stretch.	Quadratus lumborum Sacrospinalis				ing butt-ocks & pressing hips	
1–10	6.7 8.9 10	Raising & lowering leg from floor to horizontal toe pointed flexed.	8 times each leg. In each position.	3. Squeeze buttock on leg lift. 4. Breathe out on the effort.	Hamstrings Gluteals.		Less	– Inc	down Reps–	Slow tempo Simply Red

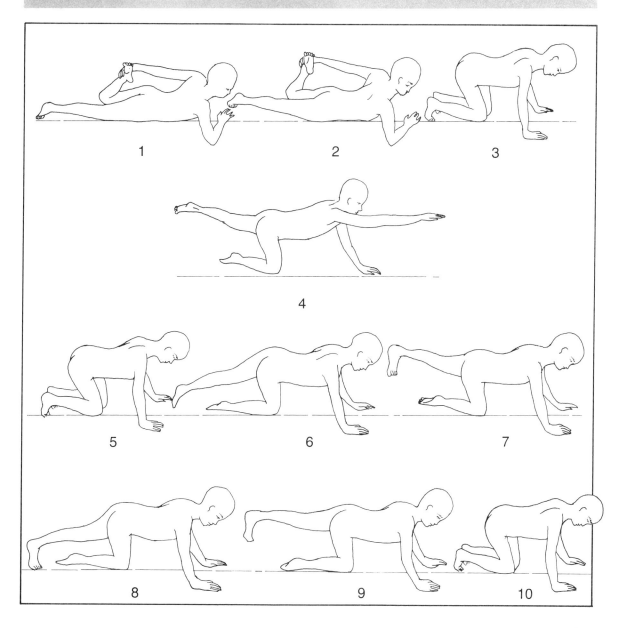

1
2
3
4
5
6
7
8
9
10

Sec	Fig no.	Activity	Sequence & Repetition	Coaching Points	Muscle Group	Fitness Component	Beg	Inter	Advan	Music
	1.	Square body position.	– 8 times. each leg.	1. Keep shoulders & hips square.	Gluteals	Muscle endurance	Less reps			As above.
D	2.3	Elbows bent low in front		2. Avoid twisting in lower back.				– Build	up reps	–
No.	4.5	Repeat wtih flexed foot.	– 8 times each leg.	3. Keep movements slow & controlled.			More release			
1–6	6.	Release in low curl.								

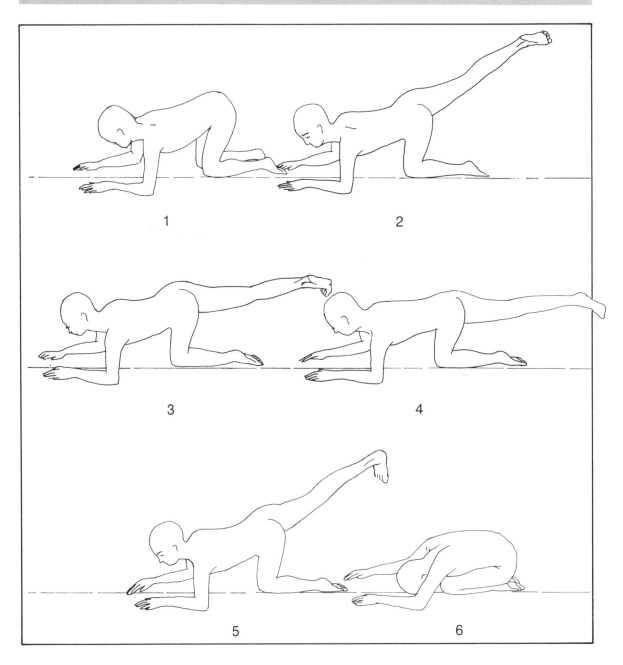

1

2

3

4

5

6

Sec	Fig no.	Activity	Sequence & Repetition	Coaching Points	Muscle Group	Fitness Component	Beg	Inter	Advan	Music
E	1.2 3	Keeping knees lifted high hips off floor Raise shoulders off floor/back	– Repeat 8 times.	1. Avoid jerking or dragging the neck.	Rectus abdominis	Muscle endurance	Less reps	–build	up reps	Slow even tempo
No.	4.5	Repeat curling elbows towards knees/ back	– Repeat 8 times	2. Breathe out on the lift up, in on the release.	Obliques	strength				Let it all blow
1–8	6.7	Twist elbow to opposite knee & release.	– Repeat 8 times							The Daz Band

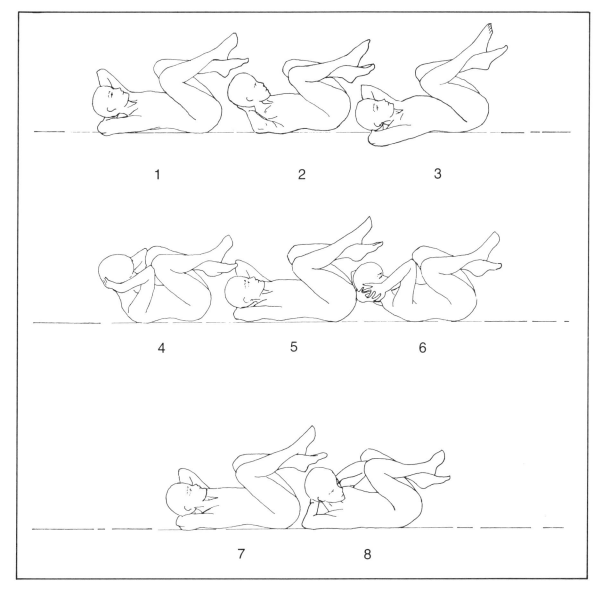

1   2   3

4   5   6

7   8

Sec	Fig no.	Activity	Sequence & Repetition	Coaching Points	Muscle Group	Fitness Component	Beg	Inter	Advan	Music
	1.2	Pelvic tilt Contract tummy muscles, press lower back to floor & tilt pelvis.	– 16 times	1. Shoulder down lengthen back of neck. Exhale on tilt Inhale on release	Hip flexors Gluteals	Muscle strength	– All	levels –		As above
F No. 1–10	3.4 5.6 7 8 9. 10.	Curl up Curl up with diagonal twist Curl up knees to release Diagonal twist knees to each side.	– 16 times – 16 times – Hold 8 counts – 8 times	2 Breathe as above Shoulders on floor knees together. Exhale as knees are lower to side.	Rectus abdominis Transversus abdominis Obliques Erector spinae		Less reps keep feet on floor	– build	up reps –	

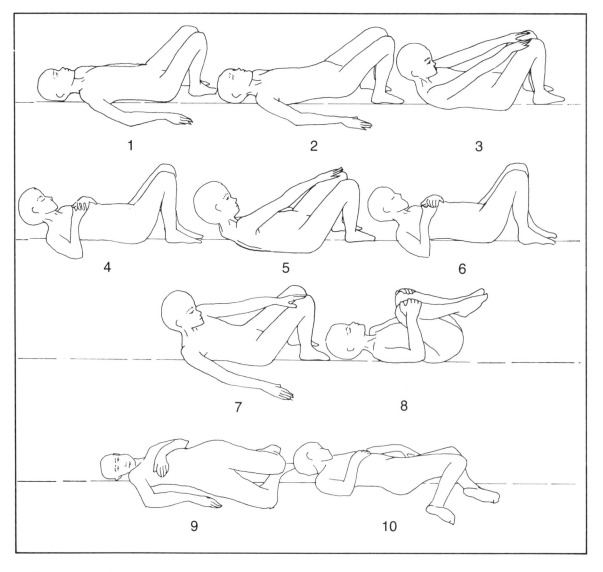

1   2   3

4   5   6

7   8

9   10

Sec	Fig no.	Activity	Sequence & Repetition	Coaching Points	Muscle Group	Fitness Component	Beg	Inter	Advan	Music
COOL DOWN		Sit tall one leg tucked sole on thigh	Hold 4 counts	1. Lift up using abdominal muscles and lower back	Latissimus dorsi					
A	2	Flat back stretch	– 8 times slowly pressing forward		Erector spinae	stretch	Think small move- ments			– inc flexibility will bring a greater stretch but this needs to be built up –
	3	Reach further	– 8 times as above	2. Release slowly forward						
No.	4	Curl over leg			Rectus abdominis					
1–6	5	Reach forward and out	8 counts	3. Curl waist backward holding abdominals tight before curling forward.	Hamstrings Hip Flexors					
	6	Lift high.	Hold 4 counts	4. Release back to reach out and lift.						

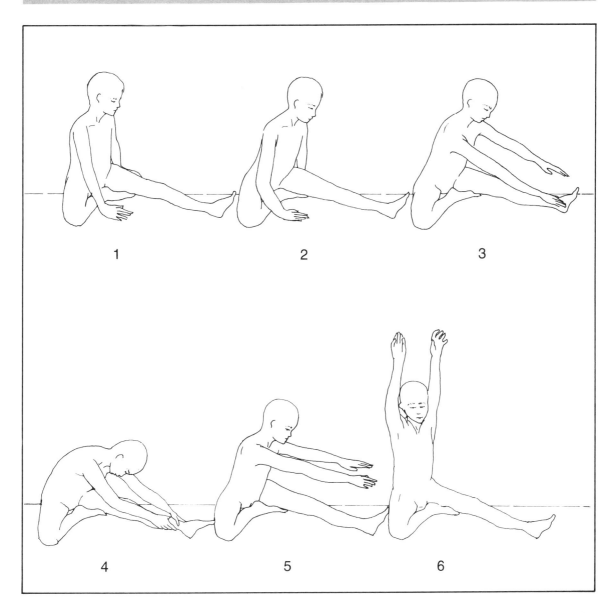

1

2

3

4

5

6

Sec	Fig no.	Activity	Sequence & Repetition	Coaching Points	Muscle Group	Fitness Component	Beg	Inter	Advan	Music
	1	Sit tall feet in front	– Hold 4 counts	1. Use abdominals & lower back muscles to hold erect.	Erector spinae Rectus abdominis		Think small move-ments	– inc flexibility will bring a greater stretch but this needs		
B	2.3	Flat back press gently forward	– 8 times slowly pressing forward		Hip flexors	Stretch		to be built up gradually.		
No. 1–6	4.	Reach further	– 8 times as above	2 Stretches should be slow and held.	Hamstrings Latissimus dorsi.					
	5.6	Curl over leg Reach forward and out Lift high	Hold 8 counts – 4 counts Hold 4 counts	3. Tuck back at waist to curl forward.				stretch		

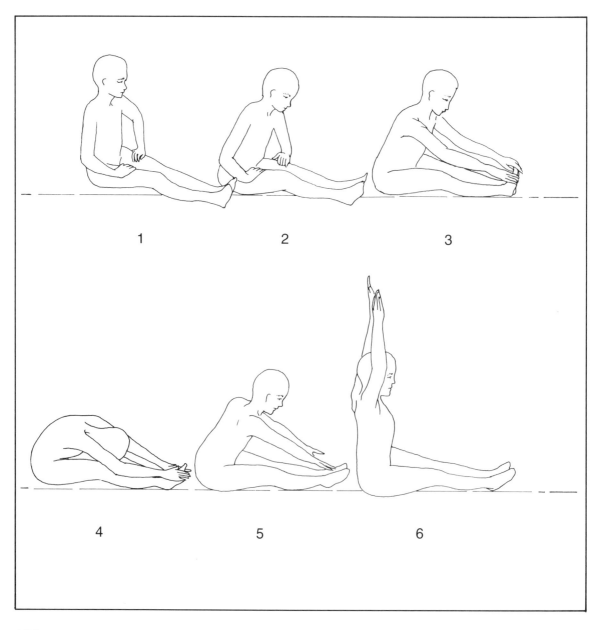

1   2   3

4   5   6

Sec	Fig no.	Activity	Sequence & Repetition	Coaching Points	Muscle Group	Fitness Component	Beg	Inter	Advan	Music
C	1.	Lying flat back, one knee bent in front on floor. Stretch other knee to chest.	eight times eight times	1. Stretches should be gentle not jerky	Hip flexors Quadriceps	Stretch		All levels		Very slow tempo
	2.	Curl up to knee	eight times in each position	2. Avoid forcing the joint into a position	Hamstrings					
No. 1-7	3.	Lying flat Straighten leg stretch foot in plantar flexion and dorsi flexion.			Inner thigh muscles					Every time we say goodbye
	4.	Rest upper leg bent across lower bent support leg Release knee out flapping gently.	eight times	3. Relax into the stretch. Exhale as thighs press down						
	5.	Raise upper leg by taking support leg off floor Press back gently.	sixteen counts	4. Press back gently. Do not force the movement	Hip	Stretch		All levels		Simply Red
	6.	Knees bent open thighs and lower out to floor.	sixteen counts							
	7.	Relax prone	Relax six seconds	take full recovery pulse – check if it is at normal resting rate						

1

2

3

4

5

6

7

Sources of Reference

Chelsea College of Physical Education, Eastbourne, Sussex. 'Human Movement Behaviour, Conference Report – Observation, Perception, Analysis. January 1975. *Journal of Human Movement Studies,* 1976.

Cooper, K., *The Aerobics Programme for Total Well Being* (Bantam, Transworld, London).

Grays Anatomy (Longmans, London).

Livingston, E. *Textbook of Physiology and Biochemistry* (Bell and Davidson).

Mosston, M., *Teaching Physical Education* (Merrill Books, Ohio).

Pearce, E.C., *Anatomy and Physiology for Nurses* (Faber & Faber, London).

Preston Dunlop, V., *A Handbook for Modern Educational Dance* (MacDonald and Evans, Plymouth, 1963).

Rowett, H.G.Q., *Basic Anatomy and Physiology* (Murray, London).

St. John Ambulance, *First Aid Manual* Dorling Kindersley, London).

Sweeney, R., *Selected Readings in Movement Education,* 1970.

Thompson, C., *Manual of Structural Kinesiology* (C.V. Mosby.)

Thompson, W.R. *Black's Medical Dictionary* (A & C Black, London).

Wirhead, R., *Athletic Ability and the Anatomy of Movement* (Wolfe Medical Publications, London).

Index